DIVERTICULITIS COOKBOOK

Healing Recipes: Safe, Delicious Nutrition for 1500 Days of Relief and Naturally Improved Health

Rosalie M. Johnson

Table of contents

CHAPTER 3: NOURISHING SOUPS AND BROTHS 51

CHAPTER 4: SALADS AND SIDES FOR GUT HEALTH 71

INTRODUCTION

In a warm kitchen filled with afternoon light, the rhythmic chop of fresh vegetables told a message of perseverance and rejuvenation.

The chef, inspired by personal experience, meticulously produced a healthy soup while reflecting on a diverticulitis journey that shaped not only meals, but also a goal to heal via food.

The struggle with diverticulitis started unexpectedly. What began as intermittent discomfort progressed to terrible pain.

Doctor visits resulted in a diagnosis and the sobering revelation that nutrition had an important role in managing this disease.

Determined to restore his health, the chef delved into the field of intestinal wellness.With each recipe perfected, the chef realized the potential of healthy components. Fiber-rich fruits and vegetables became allies, soothing broths brought comfort, and thoughtful cooking provided relief.

The kitchen was transformed into a sanctuary, with flavors and procedures that nourished the body while also lifting spirits.

However, this journey was not alone. Friends and relatives crowded around, both interested and encouraging.

They, too, sought to learn and adapt, eagerly embracing new culinary innovations. The concept of a cookbook arose from shared experiences: a compilation of recipes not just for one, but for everyone navigating the ups and downs of digestive health.

This cookbook is more than just a collection of recipes; it demonstrates the transformational power of food. Each recipe in these pages has been carefully prepared to reflect a journey - from suffering to purpose, from ambiguity to insight.

May your culinary experience provide you with inspiration and sustenance. May you discover the pleasure of cooking with intention, relishing each meal as a step towards recovery.

Whether you're starting your own path or helping a loved one, let this cookbook be your guide to the healing table, a place where health and happiness intersect, one delicious dish at a time.

Welcome to The Diverticulitis Cookbook. Let's cook our way to wellness together!

Understanding Diverticulitis

Diverticulitis is a disorder that affects many people, although its causes are often unknown. Imagine your body as a highly tuned instrument, with the digestive system conducting a complex symphony of operations.

Consider this melody broken by the presence of small pouches called diverticula that occur along the walls of the colon. These pouches, which are normally harmless, might become inflamed or infected, resulting in the development of diverticulitis.

What causes the pouches to form? It is a combination of factors, including the natural aging process and dietary decisions.Low-fiber diets, which are typical in modern lifestyles, can promote the formation of diverticula by putting strain on the colon during digestion. As the colon works harder to filter insufficient fiber, pressure builds up, resulting in weak places in its walls.

The progression from diverticula to diverticulitis is not unavoidable, but is impacted by a variety of events. Consider these pouches to be ticking time bombs, waiting for the right mix of variables - such as constipation, straining during bowel movements, or bacterial imbalance - to cause inflammation or infection.

Diverticulitis symptoms can be concerning, ranging from chronic stomach pain and soreness to fever and changes in bowel patterns. Understanding these signals is critical because fast medical attention can prevent complications such as abscesses or perforations, which require immediate treatment.

Diverticulitis is often diagnosed using a combination of clinical examination and diagnostic testing such as CT scans or colonoscopies. Patients who have received a diagnosis engage on a management path, which frequently begins with dietary changes. The cornerstone of diverticulitis treatment? Fiber is the unsung hero of intestinal health. Adequate fiber consumption regulates bowel motions and reduces constipation, which lowers the risk of diverticula formation.

What is Diverticulitis?

Diverticulitis is a digestive ailment in which tiny, bulging pouches (known as diverticula) in the lining of the colon (large intestine) become inflamed or infected.

These pouches usually occur when weak places in the colon wall give way under pressure, resulting in the creation of diverticula. Diverticula are normally innocuous and do not produce symptoms; but, when they become inflamed or infected, they can lead to diverticulitis.

The specific etiology of diverticulitis is not fully understood, however it is assumed to be associated to various variables, including:

A low-fiber diet can lead to constipation, which raises pressure within the colon during bowel movements. This increased pressure may lead to the development of diverticula.

Diverticulitis is more frequent in older persons, most likely due to the colon wall's natural weakening with age.

Genetics: Certain people may be predisposed to developing diverticula and, as a result, diverticulitis.

Diverticulitis symptoms might vary, however they often include:

Abdominal pain is often felt on the lower left side of the abdomen, although it can also occur on the right side or across the abdomen.

Tenderness: The abdomen may feel tender to the touch, particularly around the afflicted area.

Fever: Inflammation or illness can cause fever.

Change in Bowel Habits: This might include constipation, diarrhea, or alternating between the two.

Nausea and vomiting: Especially if the condition is serious.

Diverticulitis is diagnosed by a physical examination, a review of symptoms, and, in many cases, imaging tests such as a CT scan or ultrasound to determine the existence and degree of inflammation or infection.

Treatment for diverticulitis is determined on the severity of symptoms and may include:

Dietary Changes: Increase your fiber intake to avoid constipation and support healthy bowel motions.

drugs include antibiotics to treat infections, pain relievers, and drugs to soothe symptoms such as cramps.

In severe cases, hospitalization and potentially surgery may be required to drain abscesses, remove afflicted portions of the colon, or treat consequences such as perforation.

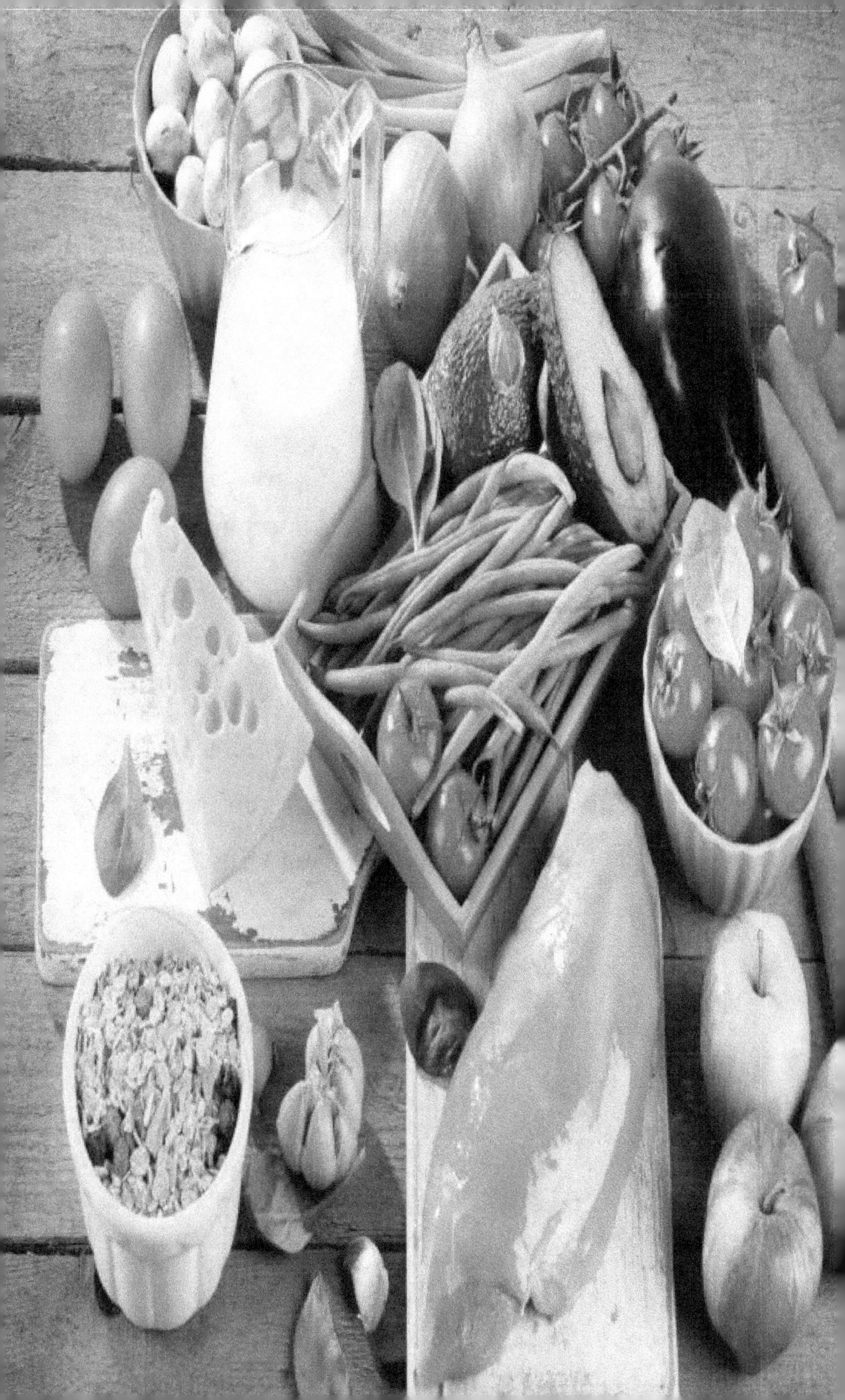

CHAPTER 1: DIET AND DIVERTICULITIS

The Role of Diet in Managing Diverticulitis

Diet is extremely important in controlling diverticulitis and lowering the risk of flare-ups. A high-fiber diet is particularly beneficial because it promotes regular bowel movements and reduces constipation, which can exacerbate diverticulitis symptoms.

Fiber-rich foods such fruits, vegetables, whole grains, and legumes should be included in meals to promote digestive health.

Furthermore, drinking sufficient of fluids, particularly water, is vital for keeping stools soft and allowing them to travel smoothly through the colon. Adequate water enhances the effectiveness of fiber in avoiding constipation.

Certain foods should be avoided or restricted to avoid exacerbating diverticulitis symptoms. These include high-fat and sugar-containing processed foods, as well as red meat and dairy products.

Spicy foods and seeds may also be avoided by certain people with diverticulitis since they can irritate the digestive system.

Foods To Eat

High-Fiber Foods: Eat plenty of berries, apples, and pears, as well as broccoli, spinach, and carrots. Fiber-rich whole grains include oats, brown rice, and quinoa.

Legumes: Beans, lentils, and chickpeas are high in fiber and protein, making them excellent meal choices.

Lean Proteins: To meet protein requirements without adding too much fat, choose lean meats such as fowl (chicken, turkey) and fish (trout, salmon).

Low-Fat Dairy: To lower your saturated fat intake, use low-fat or nonfat dairy products such yogurt and cheese.

Healthy Fats: Consume avocados, nuts, and seeds in moderation.

Hydration: Drink plenty of water throughout the day to keep your stools soft and help digestion.

Foods to avoid or limit:

Processed Foods: Avoid foods heavy in fat, sugar, and preservatives.

Limit your diet of red meat, as it can be difficult to digest and may contribute to inflammation.

Spicy meals: Some people with diverticulitis find that spicy foods aggravate their symptoms and should be avoided.

Seeds and Nuts: While opinions differ, some people may need to avoid seeds and nuts because they can clog diverticular apertures.

High-FODMAP Foods: Some high-FODMAP foods, such as onions, garlic, and some fruits, might cause bloating or discomfort in sensitive people.

Importance of Fiber

Fiber is essential for controlling diverticulitis and maintaining overall digestive health. It is critical for keeping regular bowel motions and avoiding constipation, which is a major role in lowering the risk of diverticulitis flares.

Soluble fiber in foods such as oats, beans, and fruits absorbs water and forms a gel-like substance in the intestines.

This softens feces and makes them easier to pass, lowering colon strain and preventing the formation of diverticula.

Insoluble fiber, which can be found in vegetables, whole grains, and wheat bran, bulks up stools and accelerates them through the digestive tract. This can assist to prevent constipation and improve regularity.

Incorporating high-fiber foods into your diet can bring several health benefits in addition to diverticulitis treatment. Fiber promotes satiety, which aids in the maintenance of good cholesterol levels, blood sugar regulation, and weight management.

To avoid pain or bloating, gradually increase your fiber intake while drinking lots of fluids. Aim for at least 25-30 grams of fiber per day from a variety of fruits, vegetables, whole grains, and legumes to promote digestive function and effectively manage diverticulitis.

This cookbook contains delicious and fiber-rich dishes to assist people with diverticulitis eat a varied and nutritious diet that promotes digestive health.

Fluid Intake

Adequate fluid consumption is critical for controlling diverticulitis and maintaining intestinal health. Adequate water softens feces, making them easier to pass and lowering the risk of constipation, which is an important component in avoiding diverticulitis flare-ups.

Water is the best option for hydration, although herbal teas, broths, and diluted fruit juices can also help with regular fluid intake. Aim to drink at least 8-10 cups (approximately 2-2.5 liters) of fluids each day, equally distributed throughout the day.

Maintaining hydration is especially crucial during acute episodes of diverticulitis because it helps the body repair and prevents complications. However, excessive caffeine and alcohol use should be avoided because they might dehydrate the body and irritate the digestive tract.

Drinking fluids with meals and snacks might also be beneficial. A bowl of clear broth-based soup, or adding sliced fruits like oranges or cucumbers to water, can help with hydration and overall dietary fiber consumption.

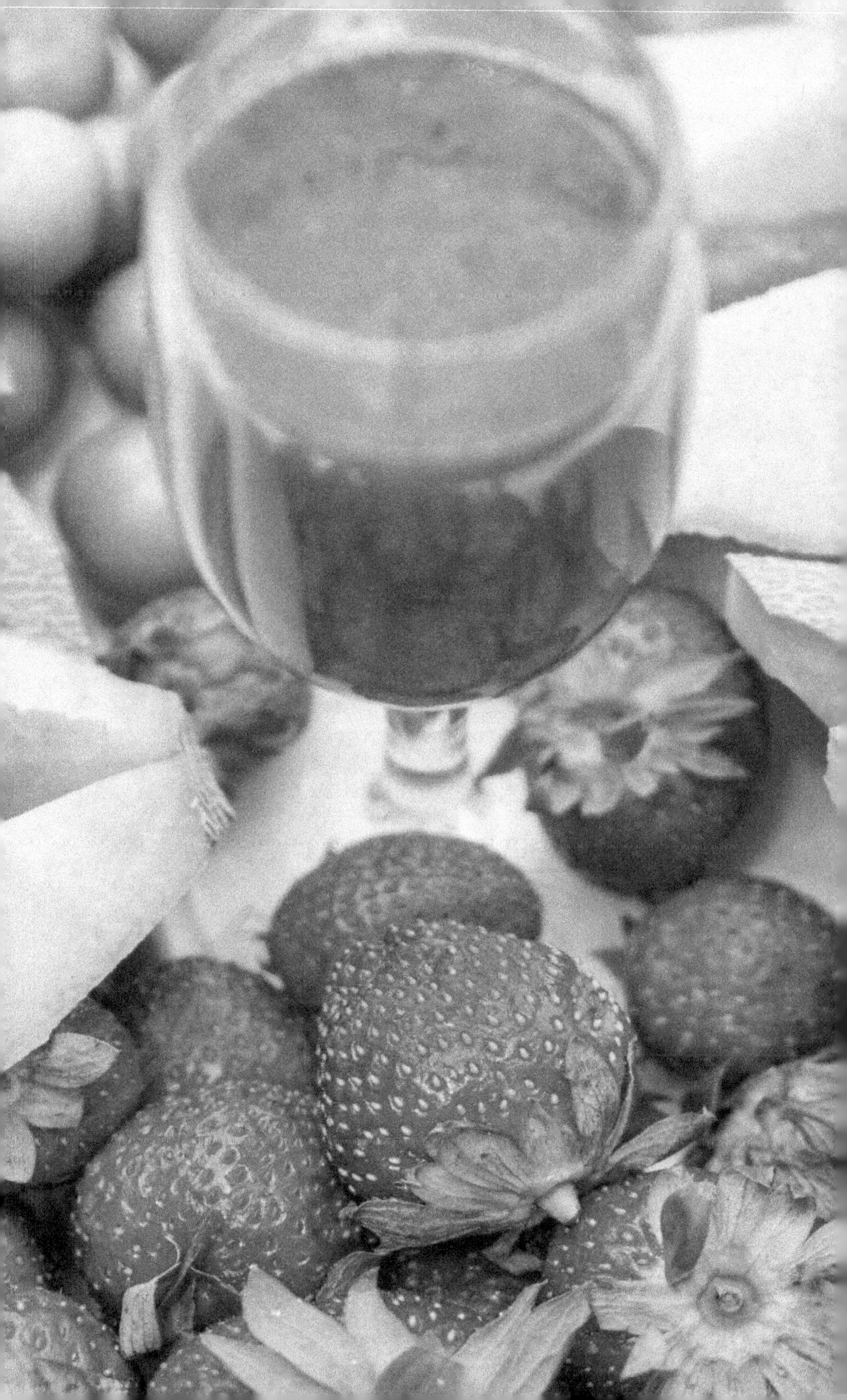

CHAPTER 2: BREAKFASTS FOR DIGESTIVE WELLNESS

Oatmeal with Berries and Chia Seeds

Ingredients:

- 1/2 cup rolled oats
- 1 cup water or almond milk
- 1/2 cup mixed berries (strawberries, blueberries, raspberries)
- 1 tablespoon chia seeds
- Optional: honey or maple syrup for sweetness

Instructions:

1. In a small saucepan, bring water or almond milk to a boil.

2. Add rolled oats and reduce heat to a simmer. Cook for 5-7 minutes, stirring occasionally, until oats are tender and creamy.

3. Remove from heat and transfer oatmeal to a bowl.

4. Top with mixed berries and sprinkle chia seeds over the berries.

5. Drizzle with honey or maple syrup if desired.

6. Enjoy warm!

Nutrient:

Calories:	Fiber:	Protein:	Fat:
300	8g	9g	5g

Greek Yogurt Parfait

Ingredients:

- 1 cup Greek yogurt (unsweetened)
- 1/2 banana, sliced
- 1/2 cup fresh strawberries, sliced
- 1/4 cup granola (low-sugar or homemade)

Instructions:

1. In a glass or bowl, layer Greek yogurt, sliced banana, and sliced strawberries.
2. Sprinkle granola on top.
3. Repeat layers if desired.
4. Serve chilled.

Nutrient:

Calories:	Fiber:	Protein:	Fat:
280	5g	20g	8g

Smoothie Bowl

Ingredients:

- 1 ripe banana
- 1 cup spinach leaves
- 1/2 cup frozen pineapple chunks
- 1/2 cup unsweetened almond milk
- Toppings: sliced almonds, shredded coconut

Instructions:

1. In a blender, combine banana, spinach, frozen pineapple, and almond milk.
2. Blend until smooth and creamy.
3. Pour into a bowl.
4. Top with sliced almonds and shredded coconut.
5. Enjoy with a spoon!

Calories:	Fiber:	Protein:	Fat: 9g
280	7g	5g	

Scrambled Eggs with Spinach

Ingredients:

- 2 eggs
- Handful of fresh spinach leaves
- Salt and pepper to taste
- Optional: 1 tablespoon shredded low-fat cheese

Instructions:

1. In a bowl, beat eggs with salt and pepper.
2. Heat a non-stick skillet over medium heat.
3. Add spinach to the skillet and cook until wilted.

4. Pour beaten eggs over the spinach.

5. Stir gently until eggs are cooked to desired consistency.

6. Sprinkle with shredded cheese if using.

7. Serve hot.

Calories:	Fiber:	Protein:	Fat:
220	2g	14g	15g

Banana Pancakes

Ingredients:

- 1 ripe banana, mashed
- 2 eggs
- 1/4 teaspoon cinnamon
- Coconut oil for cooking

1. In a bowl, mash the banana until smooth.
2. Add eggs and cinnamon to the mashed banana. Mix until well combined.
3. Heat a non-stick skillet over medium heat and lightly grease with coconut oil.
4. Pour small portions of the batter onto the skillet to form pancakes.
5. Cook for 2-3 minutes on each side, or until golden brown.
6. Serve warm with a side of fresh fruit.

Nutrient:

Calories:	Fiber:	Protein:	Fat:
250	3g	10g	10g

Quinoa Breakfast Bowl

Ingredients:

- 1/2 cup cooked quinoa
- 1/2 peach, sliced
- 1 tablespoon slivered almonds
- 1 tablespoon honey

Instructions:

1. In a bowl, layer cooked quinoa with sliced peach.
2. Top with slivered almonds.
3. Drizzle with honey.
4. Serve warm or chilled.

Nutrient:

Calories:	Fiber:	Protein:	Fat:
280	5g	8g	5g

Chia Seed Pudding

Ingredients:

- 2 tablespoons chia seeds
- 1/2 cup unsweetened almond milk
- 1/2 cup mango puree
- Optional toppings: sliced kiwi, Greek yogurt

Instructions:

1. In a bowl, mix chia seeds and almond milk.
2. Let it sit for 10 minutes, then stir again to break up any clumps.
3. Refrigerate for at least 1 hour or overnight until thickened.
4. Layer chia pudding with mango puree in a glass.
5. Top with sliced kiwi and a dollop of Greek yogurt if desired.
6. Enjoy chilled.

Calories:	Fiber:	Protein:	Fat:
220	12g	6g	10g

Whole Grain Toast with Avocado

Ingredients:

- 1 slice whole grain toast
- 1/4 ripe avocado, mashed
- Pinch of sea salt
- Optional: pumpkin seeds for topping

Instructions:

1. Toast a slice of whole grain bread until golden.
2. Spread mashed avocado on top.
3. Sprinkle with a pinch of sea salt.
4. Garnish with pumpkin seeds if desired.

5. Serve immediately.

Calories:	Fiber:	Protein:	Fat:
180	5g	4g	8g

Berry Smoothie

Ingredients:

- 1/2 cup mixed berries (strawberries, blueberries, raspberries)
- Handful of spinach leaves
- 1/2 cup unsweetened Greek yogurt
- 1/2 cup water or almond milk

Instructions:

1. In a blender, combine mixed berries, spinach, Greek yogurt, and water/almond milk.
2. Blend until smooth and creamy.

3. Pour into a glass and serve
   immediately.

Calories:	Fiber:	Protein:	Fat:
180	5g	15g	4g

Apple Cinnamon Baked Oatmeal

Ingredients:

- 1 cup rolled oats
- 1 apple, diced
- 1 teaspoon cinnamon
- 1 tablespoon honey
- 1 cup almond milk

1. Preheat the oven to 350°F (175°C).

2. In a bowl, mix rolled oats, diced apple, cinnamon, honey, and almond milk.

3. Transfer mixture to a baking dish.

4. Bake for 25-30 minutes until oats are cooked and apples are tender.

5. Remove from the oven and let it cool slightly before serving.

6. Divide into portions and enjoy warm.

Nutrient:

Calories:	Fiber:	Protein:	Fat: 4g
280	6g	7g	

Egg and Veggie Muffin Cups

Ingredients:

- 4 eggs
- 1/2 cup chopped bell peppers (red, green, yellow)
- 1 cup chopped spinach
- Salt and pepper to taste
- Optional: 2 tablespoons crumbled feta cheese

Instructions:

1. Preheat the oven to 350°F (175°C) and grease a muffin tin.
2. In a bowl, beat eggs with salt and pepper.
3. Stir in chopped bell peppers and spinach.
4. Pour egg mixture into each muffin cup, filling about 3/4 full.
5. Sprinkle crumbled feta cheese on top if using.

6. Bake for 15-18 minutes until eggs are set and lightly golden.

7. Allow to cool slightly before removing from the muffin tin.

8. Serve warm or refrigerate for later.

Nutrient :

Calories: 120 (per muffin)	Fiber: 2g	Protein: 8g	Fat: 7g

Overnight Buckwheat Porridge

Ingredients:

- 1/2 cup raw buckwheat groats
- 1 cup almond milk
- 1/4 cup chopped nuts (walnuts, almonds)
- 2 tablespoons dried apricots, chopped

- 1 tablespoon honey

Instructions:

1. Rinse buckwheat groats under cold water and drain well.
2. In a bowl, combine buckwheat groats, almond milk, chopped nuts, dried apricots, and honey.
3. Cover and refrigerate overnight.
4. In the morning, stir well and add more almond milk if desired for desired consistency.
5. Serve cold or warmed up.

Nutrient:

Calories:	Fiber:	Protein:	Fat:
320	8g	10g	15g

Mango Coconut Chia Pudding

Ingredients:

- 3 tablespoons chia seeds
- 1/2 cup coconut milk
- 1/2 cup mango puree (fresh or frozen)
- Optional: sliced kiwi for garnish

Instructions:

1. In a bowl, mix chia seeds and coconut milk.
2. Let it sit for 10 minutes, then stir again to break up any clumps.
3. In a separate bowl, blend fresh or frozen mango into a puree.
4. Layer chia pudding with mango puree in a glass or bowl.
5. Garnish with sliced kiwi if desired.

6. Chill in the refrigerator for at least 1
    hour before serving.

Calories:	Fiber:	Protein:	Fat:
250	10g	6g	15g

Spinach and Feta Omelette

Ingredients:

- 2 eggs
- Handful of fresh spinach leaves
- 2 tablespoons crumbled feta cheese
- Salt and pepper to taste

Instructions:

1. In a bowl, beat eggs with salt and
    pepper.

2. Heat a non-stick skillet over
   medium heat.
3. Add fresh spinach to the skillet and
   cook until wilted.
4. Pour beaten eggs over the spinach.
5. Sprinkle crumbled feta cheese on
   top.
6. Cook until eggs are set and cheese
   is melted.
7. Fold omelette in half and slide onto
   a plate.
8. Serve hot with a side of whole grain
   toast.

Nutrient:

Calories:	Fiber:	Protein:	Fat:
250	2g	14g	18g

Cottage Cheese Bowl

Ingredients:

- 1/2 cup low-fat cottage cheese
- 1/2 cup sliced peaches (fresh or canned in juice)
- 1 tablespoon sunflower seeds
- Optional: drizzle of honey

Instructions:

1. In a bowl, combine cottage cheese and sliced peaches.
2. Top with sunflower seeds.
3. Drizzle with honey if desired.
4. Enjoy as is or with a slice of whole grain toast.

Nutrient:

Calories:	Fiber:	Protein:	Fat:
200	3g	15g	8g

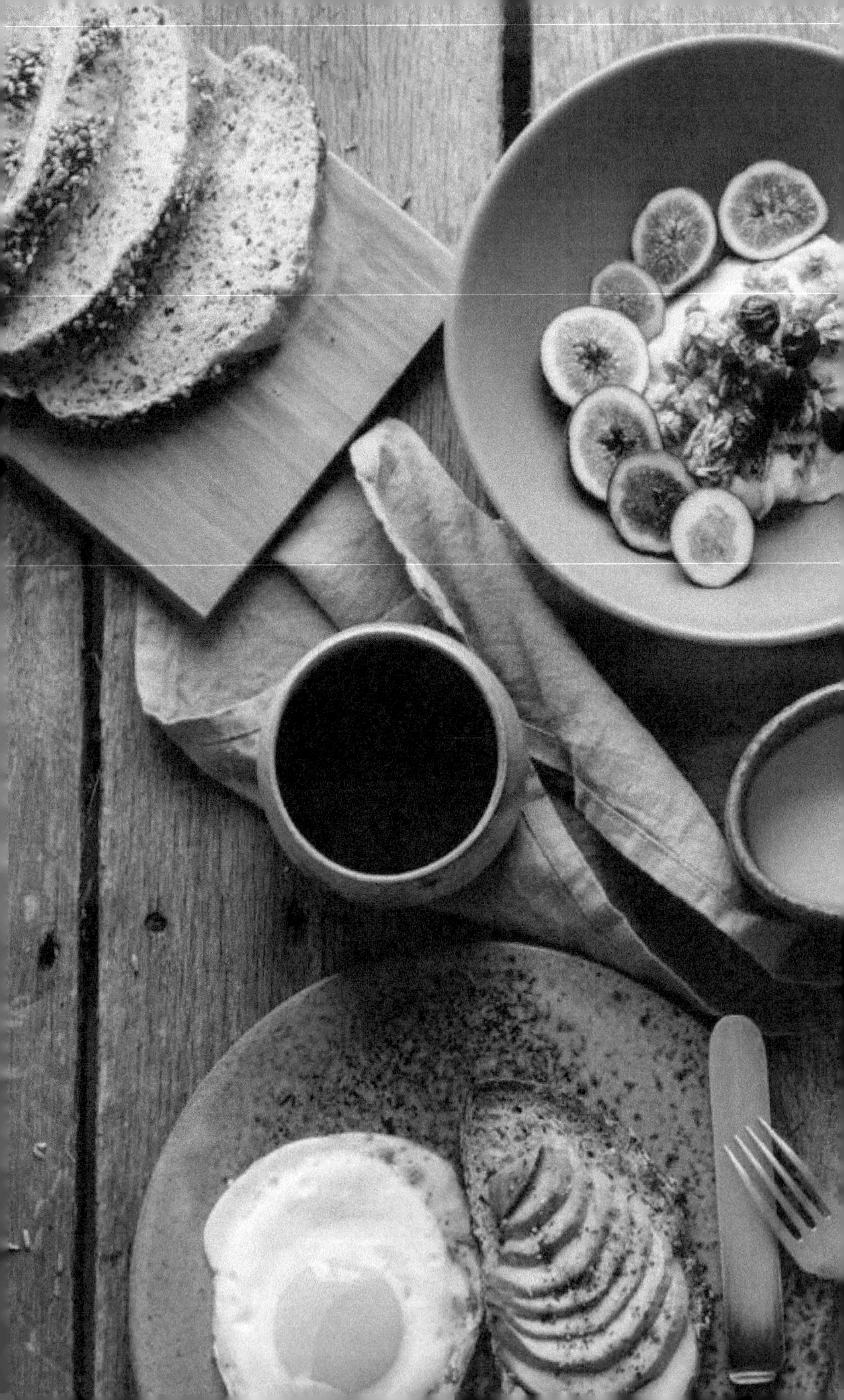

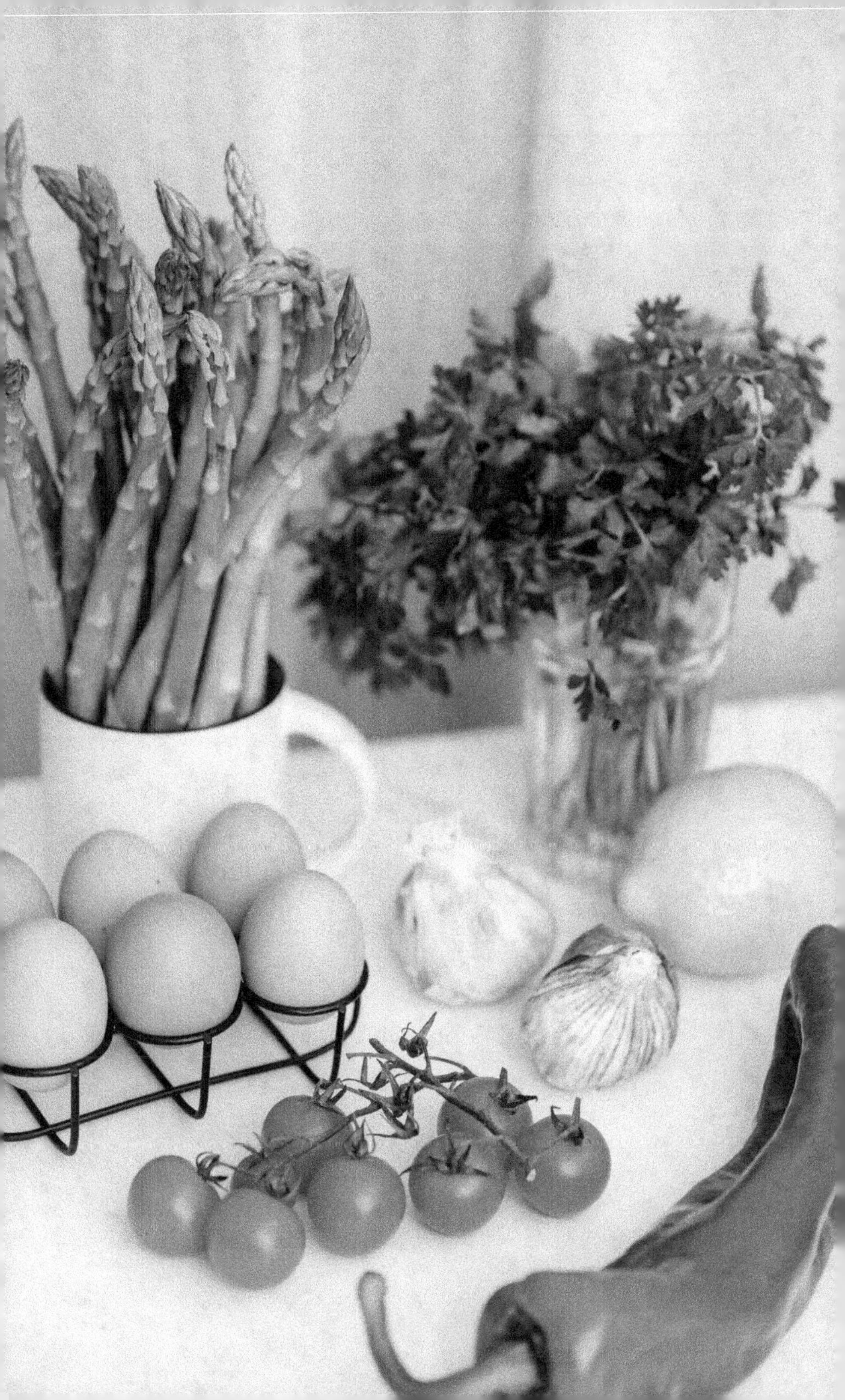

CHAPTER 3:
NOURISHING SOUPS AND BROTHS

Chicken and Vegetable Soup

Ingredients:

- 1 tablespoon olive oil
- 1 onion, chopped
- 2 carrots, sliced
- 2 celery stalks, diced
- 2 cloves garlic, minced
- 4 cups low-sodium chicken broth
- 2 cups cooked shredded chicken breast
- Salt and pepper to taste
- Fresh parsley for garnish

1. Heat olive oil in a large pot over medium heat.
2. Add chopped onion, carrots, celery, and garlic. Sauté until vegetables are tender, about 5-7 minutes.
3. Pour in chicken broth and bring to a simmer.
4. Add shredded chicken and simmer for another 10-15 minutes.
5. Season with salt and pepper to taste.
6. Serve hot, garnished with fresh parsley.

Nutrient:

Calories:	Fiber:	Protein:	Fat: 8g
200	3g	20g	

Lentil Soup

Ingredients:

- 1 tablespoon olive oil
- 1 onion, chopped
- 2 carrots, diced
- 2 celery stalks, diced
- 1 cup dried green lentils, rinsed
- 4 cups vegetable broth
- 1 bay leaf
- Salt and pepper to taste
- Fresh parsley for garnish

Instructions:

1. Heat olive oil in a pot over medium heat.
2. Add chopped onion, carrots, and celery. Sauté until vegetables soften, about 5 minutes.

3. Stir in dried lentils, vegetable broth,
    and bay leaf.

4. Bring to a boil, then reduce heat and
    simmer for 20-25 minutes until
    lentils are tender.

5. Season with salt and pepper to taste.

6. Remove bay leaf before serving.

7. Garnish with fresh parsley.

Nutrient:

Calories:	Fiber:	Protein:	Fat: 5g
250	12g	14g	

Butternut Squash Soup

Ingredients:

- 1 butternut squash, peeled, seeded, and diced
- 1 onion, chopped
- 2 carrots, diced
- 2 celery stalks, diced
- 4 cups low-sodium vegetable broth
- 1 teaspoon ground cinnamon
- Salt and pepper to taste
- Optional: Greek yogurt for garnish

Instructions:

1. In a large pot, combine diced butternut squash, onion, carrots, celery, and vegetable broth.
2. Bring to a boil, then reduce heat and simmer for 20-25 minutes until vegetables are tender.

3. Use an immersion blender to puree the soup until smooth.

4. Stir in ground cinnamon, salt, and pepper.

5. Serve hot, optionally topped with a dollop of Greek yogurt.

Nutrient:

Calories:	Fiber:	Protein:	Fat: 1g
180	6g	4g	

Tomato Basil Soup

Ingredients:

- 1 tablespoon olive oil
- 1 onion, chopped
- 2 cloves garlic, minced
- 1 can (28 oz) crushed tomatoes
- 4 cups low-sodium vegetable broth
- 1/4 cup chopped fresh basil

- Salt and pepper to taste
- Optional: grated Parmesan cheese for garnish

Instructions:

1. Heat olive oil in a pot over medium heat.
2. Add chopped onion and minced garlic. Sauté until onion becomes translucent, about 5 minutes.
3. Stir in crushed tomatoes and vegetable broth.
4. Simmer for 15-20 minutes.
5. Add chopped fresh basil, salt, and pepper.
6. Use an immersion blender to blend until smooth.
7. Serve hot, garnished with grated Parmesan cheese if desired.

Nutrient

Calories: 150	Fiber: 5g	Protein: 4g	Fat: 5g

Chicken Bone Broth

Ingredients:

- 2-3 pounds chicken bones (such as carcass or wings)
- 1 onion, quartered
- 2 carrots, chopped
- 2 celery stalks, chopped
- 2 garlic cloves, smashed
- 1 tablespoon apple cider vinegar
- Water, enough to cover the ingredients
- Salt and pepper to taste

1. Place chicken bones, onion, carrots, celery, garlic, and apple cider vinegar in a large stockpot.

2. Add enough water to cover the ingredients.

3. Bring to a boil, then reduce heat to low and simmer for 12-24 hours, skimming off any foam that rises to the top.

4. Strain the broth through a fine-mesh sieve or cheesecloth.

5. Season with salt and pepper to taste.

6. Use immediately or store in the refrigerator for up to 5 days or freeze for longer storage.

Nutrient :

Calories:	Protein:	Fat:
40 (per cup)	6g	2g

Vegetable Miso Soup

Ingredients:

- 4 cups vegetable broth
- 1 tablespoon miso paste
- 1 cup sliced mushrooms (shiitake, button, or mixed)
- 1 block tofu, diced
- 2 green onions, thinly sliced
- 1 tablespoon soy sauce or tamari
- Optional: seaweed (such as nori or wakame) for garnish

1. In a pot, bring vegetable broth to a simmer.
2. In a small bowl, dissolve miso paste in a ladleful of hot broth.
3. Add dissolved miso paste back to the pot.
4. Add sliced mushrooms and diced tofu.
5. Simmer for 5-7 minutes until mushrooms are tender.
6. Stir in sliced green onions and soy sauce.
7. Serve hot, garnished with seaweed if desired.

Nutrient:

Calories:	Fiber:	Protein:	Fat: 5g
120	3g	10g	

Creamy Broccoli Soup

Ingredients

- 1 tablespoon olive oil
- 1 onion, chopped
- 2 cloves garlic, minced
- 4 cups chopped broccoli florets
- 4 cups low-sodium vegetable broth
- 1/2 cup unsweetened almond milk
- Salt and pepper to taste
- Optional: grated cheddar cheese for garnish

Instructions:

1. Heat olive oil in a pot over medium heat.
2. Add chopped onion and minced garlic. Sauté until onion becomes translucent, about 5 minutes.

3. Add chopped broccoli florets and vegetable broth to the pot.

4. Bring to a simmer and cook for 15-20 minutes until broccoli is tender.

5. Use an immersion blender to puree the soup until smooth.

6. Stir in unsweetened almond milk.

7. Season with salt and pepper to taste.

8. Serve hot, optionally topped with grated cheddar cheese.

Nutrient :

Calories:	Fiber:	Protein:	Fat:
180	5g	7g	9g

Split Pea Soup

Ingredients:

- 1 tablespoon olive oil
- 1 onion, chopped
- 2 carrots, diced
- 2 celery stalks, diced
- 1 cup dried split green peas, rinsed
- 4 cups vegetable broth
- 1 bay leaf
- Salt and pepper to taste

Instructions:

1. Heat olive oil in a pot over medium heat.
2. Add chopped onion, carrots, and celery. Sauté until vegetables soften, about 5 minutes.
3. Stir in dried split green peas and vegetable broth.

4. Add bay leaf.

5. Bring to a boil, then reduce heat and simmer for 45-60 minutes until peas are tender.

6. Remove bay leaf before serving.

7. Season with salt and pepper to taste.

8. Serve hot.

Nutrient:

Calories:	Fiber:	Protein:	Fat: 4g
220	12g	9g	

Creamy Potato Leek Soup

Ingredients:

- 2 tablespoons butter or olive oil
- 2 leeks, white and light green parts only, sliced
- 3 potatoes, peeled and diced
- 4 cups low-sodium vegetable broth

- 1 cup unsweetened almond milk
- Salt and pepper to taste
- Chopped fresh chives for garnish

Instructions:

1. In a pot, melt butter or heat olive oil over medium heat.
2. Add sliced leeks and sauté until softened, about 5 minutes.
3. Add diced potatoes and vegetable broth to the pot.
4. Bring to a simmer and cook for 15-20 minutes until potatoes are tender.
5. Use an immersion blender to puree the soup until smooth.
6. Stir in unsweetened almond milk.
7. Season with salt and pepper to taste.
8. Serve hot, garnished with chopped fresh chives.

Calories:	Fiber:	Protein:	Fat:
250	5g	5g	8g

Turmeric Ginger Carrot Soup

Ingredients:

- 1 tablespoon olive oil
- 1 onion, chopped
- 2 cloves garlic, minced
- 1 tablespoon grated fresh ginger
- 1 teaspoon ground turmeric
- 4 cups chopped carrots
- 4 cups low-sodium vegetable broth
- Salt and pepper to taste
- Fresh cilantro for garnish

1. Heat olive oil in a pot over medium heat.

2. Add chopped onion, minced garlic, grated ginger, and ground turmeric. Sauté until fragrant, about 2 minutes.

3. Add chopped carrots and vegetable broth to the pot.

4. Bring to a simmer and cook for 20-25 minutes until carrots are tender.

5. Use an immersion blender to puree the soup until smooth.

6. Season with salt and pepper to taste.

7. Serve hot, garnished with fresh cilantro.

Nutrient:

Calories:	Fiber:	Protein:	Fat:
180	6g	4g	6g

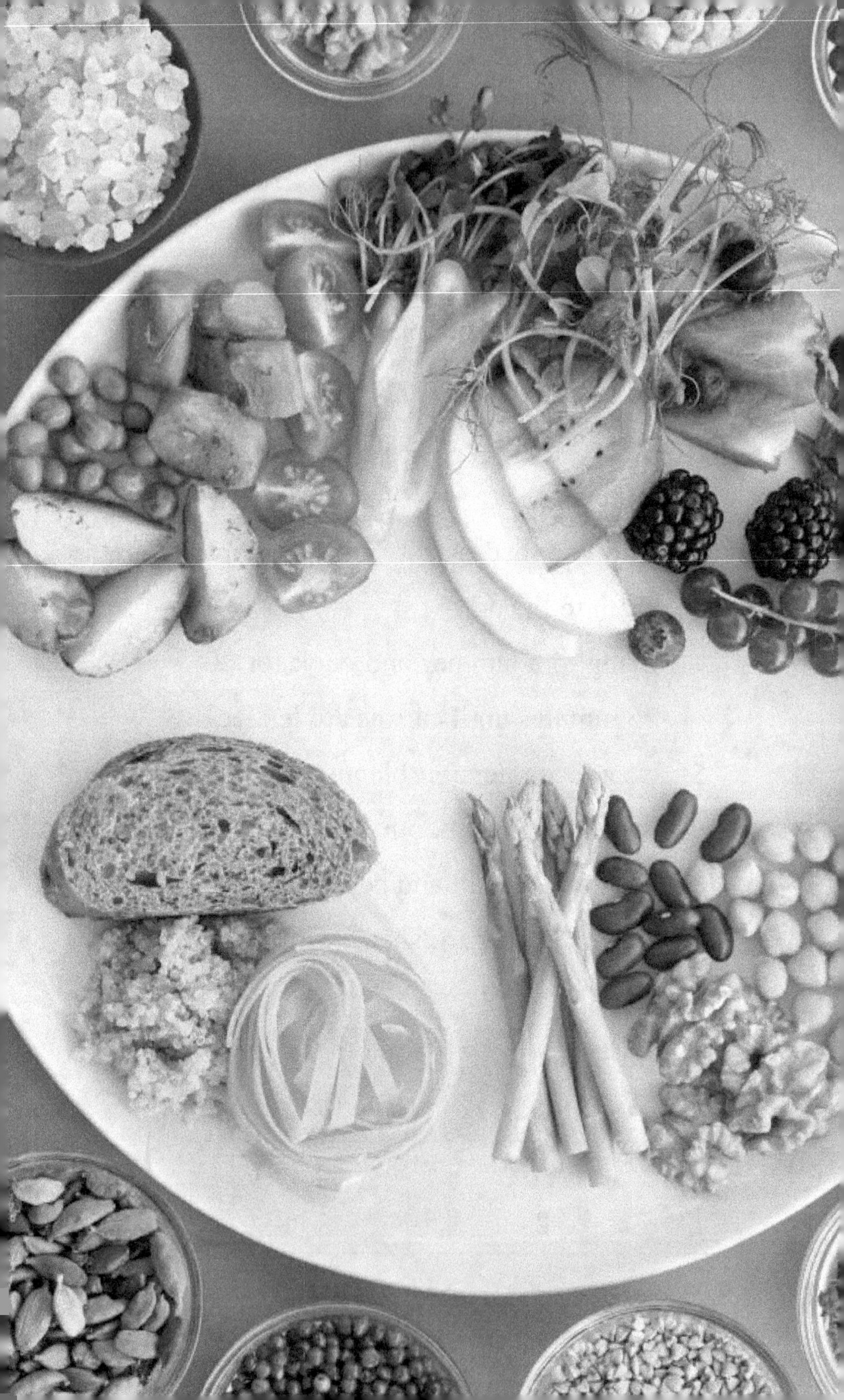

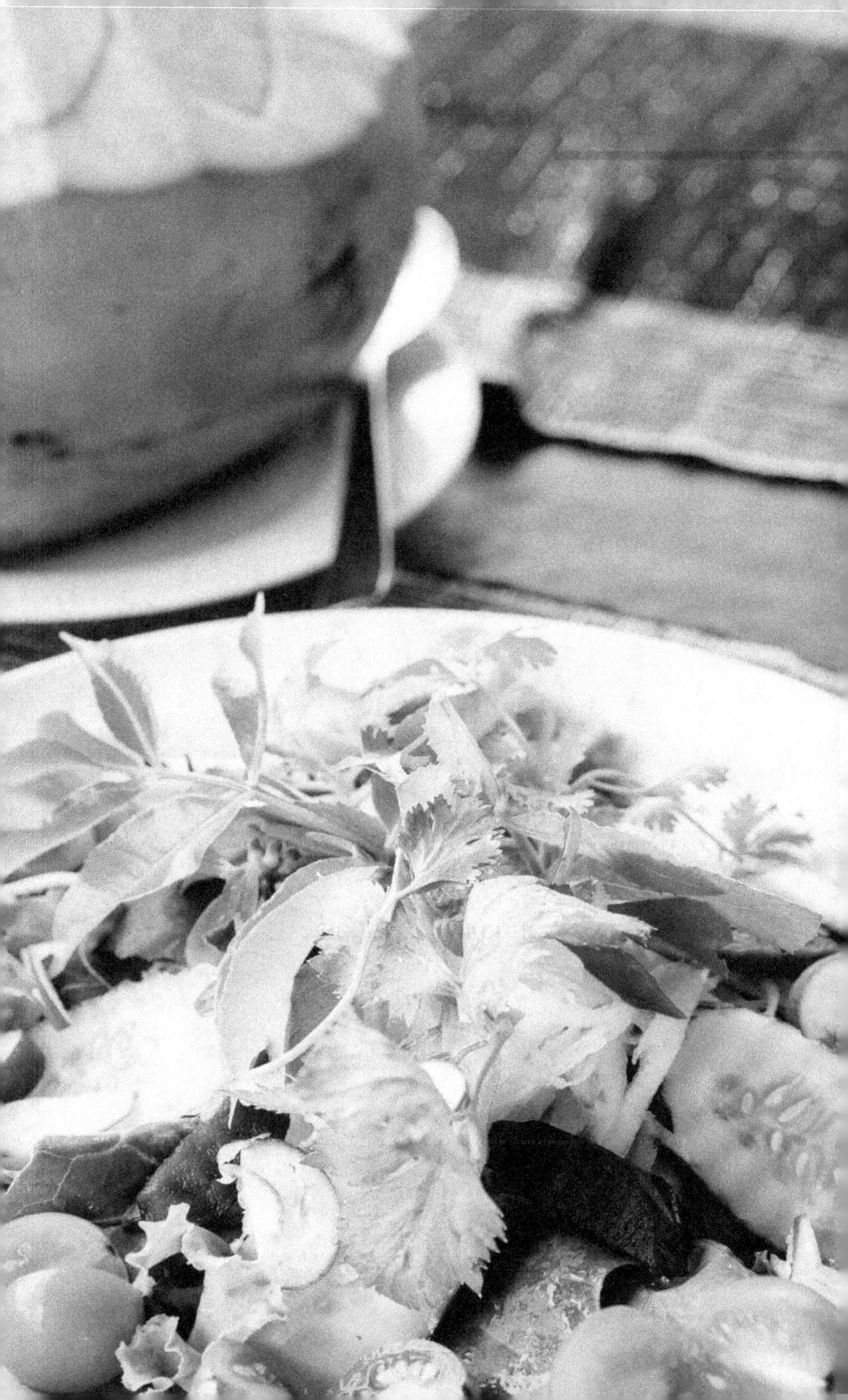

CHAPTER 4: SALADS AND SIDES FOR GUT HEALTH

Quinoa Salad with Roasted Vegetables

Ingredients:

- 1 cup cooked quinoa
- 1 zucchini, sliced
- 1 red bell pepper, sliced
- 1 small eggplant, diced
- 2 tablespoons olive oil
- Salt and pepper to taste
- Fresh parsley, chopped

Instructions:

1. Preheat the oven to 400°F (200°C).

2. Toss sliced zucchini, red bell pepper, and diced eggplant with olive oil, salt, and pepper.

3. Spread the vegetables on a baking sheet and roast for 20-25 minutes until tender and slightly browned.

4. In a large bowl, combine cooked quinoa with roasted vegetables.

5. Drizzle with additional olive oil if desired.

6. Season with salt and pepper to taste.

7. Garnish with fresh chopped parsley.

8. Serve warm or chilled.

Nutrient:

Calories:	Fiber:	Protein:	Fat: 9g
220	6g	5g	

Greek Chickpea Salad

Ingredients:

- 1 can (15 oz) chickpeas, drained and rinsed
- 1 cucumber, diced
- 1 cup cherry tomatoes, halved
- 1/4 red onion, thinly sliced
- 1/4 cup crumbled feta cheese
- 2 tablespoons olive oil
- 1 tablespoon red wine vinegar
- 1 teaspoon dried oregano
- Salt and pepper to taste

Instructions:

1. In a large bowl, combine chickpeas, diced cucumber, cherry tomatoes, sliced red onion, and crumbled feta cheese.

2. In a small bowl, whisk together olive oil, red wine vinegar, dried oregano, salt, and pepper.

3. Pour the dressing over the salad and toss to combine.

4. Adjust seasoning if needed.

5. Serve chilled as a refreshing side dish or light lunch.

Nutrient:

Calories:	Fiber:	Protein:	Fat:
280	8g	9g	14g

Spinach Salad with Strawberries and Almonds

Ingredients:

- 4 cups fresh spinach leaves
- 1 cup sliced strawberries
- 1/4 cup sliced almonds

- 2 tablespoons balsamic vinegar
- 1 tablespoon olive oil
- 1 teaspoon honey
- Salt and pepper to taste

Instructions:

1. In a large bowl, combine fresh spinach leaves, sliced strawberries, and sliced almonds.
2. In a small bowl, whisk together balsamic vinegar, olive oil, honey, salt, and pepper.
3. Drizzle the dressing over the salad and toss gently to coat.
4. Serve immediately as a vibrant and nutritious side dish.

Nutrient;

Calories:	Fiber:	Protein:	Fat:
180	5g	5g	12g

Cabbage and Carrot Slaw

Ingredients:

- 3 cups shredded green cabbage
- 1 cup shredded carrots
- 1/4 cup chopped fresh parsley
- 2 tablespoons olive oil
- 2 tablespoons apple cider vinegar
- 1 teaspoon Dijon mustard
- Salt and pepper to taste

Instructions:

1. In a large bowl, combine shredded green cabbage, shredded carrots, and chopped fresh parsley.

2. In a small bowl, whisk together olive oil, apple cider vinegar, Dijon mustard, salt, and pepper.

3. Pour the dressing over the cabbage mixture and toss to combine.

4. Refrigerate for at least 30 minutes before serving to allow flavors to meld.

5. Serve chilled as a crunchy and tangy side salad.

Calories:	Fiber:	Protein:	Fat:
120	4g	2g	8g

Mediterranean Quinoa Salad

Ingredients:

- 1 cup cooked quinoa
- 1 cucumber, diced
- 1 cup cherry tomatoes, halved
- 1/4 red onion, thinly sliced
- 1/4 cup pitted Kalamata olives, halved
- 2 tablespoons crumbled feta cheese

- 2 tablespoons olive oil
- 1 tablespoon lemon juice
- 1 teaspoon dried oregano
- Salt and pepper to taste

Instructions:

1. In a large bowl, combine cooked quinoa, diced cucumber, cherry tomatoes, sliced red onion, halved Kalamata olives, and crumbled feta cheese.
2. In a small bowl, whisk together olive oil, lemon juice, dried oregano, salt, and pepper.
3. Drizzle the dressing over the salad and toss to combine.
4. Adjust seasoning if needed.
5. Serve chilled as a satisfying and flavorful salad.

Nutrient:

Calories:	Fiber:	Protein:	Fat:
250	6g	7g	14g

Roasted Beet and Goat Cheese Salad

Ingredients:

- 2 medium beets, roasted, peeled, and sliced
- 4 cups mixed salad greens (such as arugula or baby spinach)
- 1/4 cup crumbled goat cheese
- 1/4 cup walnuts, toasted
- 2 tablespoons balsamic vinegar
- 1 tablespoon olive oil
- Salt and pepper to taste

1. Preheat the oven to 400°F (200°C). Wrap beets in foil and roast for 45-60 minutes until tender. Let cool, then peel and slice.

2. In a large bowl, combine mixed salad greens, roasted beet slices, crumbled goat cheese, and toasted walnuts.

3. In a small bowl, whisk together balsamic vinegar, olive oil, salt, and pepper.

4. Drizzle the dressing over the salad and toss gently to coat.

5. Serve immediately as a colorful and nutritious side salad.

Nutrient:

Calories:	Fiber:	Protein:	Fat:
220	4g	7g	16g

Cucumber Tomato Salad

Ingredients:

- 2 cucumbers, sliced
- 2 cups cherry tomatoes, halved
- 1/4 red onion, thinly sliced
- 2 tablespoons chopped fresh dill
- 2 tablespoons olive oil
- 1 tablespoon red wine vinegar
- Salt and pepper to taste

Instructions:

1. In a large bowl, combine sliced cucumbers, halved cherry tomatoes, thinly sliced red onion, and chopped fresh dill.
2. In a small bowl, whisk together olive oil, red wine vinegar, salt, and pepper.

3. Drizzle the dressing over the salad and toss gently to combine.

4. Refrigerate for at least 30 minutes before serving to enhance flavors.

5. Serve chilled as a crisp and refreshing side salad.

Nutrient:

Calories:	Fiber:	Protein:	Fat:
120	3g	2g	9g

Broccoli Salad with Cranberries and Almonds

Ingredients:

- 4 cups chopped broccoli florets
- 1/4 cup dried cranberries
- 1/4 cup sliced almonds
- 1/4 red onion, thinly sliced
- 1/4 cup plain Greek yogurt

- 2 tablespoons mayonnaise
- 1 tablespoon apple cider vinegar
- 1 teaspoon honey
- Salt and pepper to taste

Instructions:

1. In a large bowl, combine chopped broccoli florets, dried cranberries, sliced almonds, and thinly sliced red onion.

2. In a small bowl, whisk together Greek yogurt, mayonnaise, apple cider vinegar, honey, salt, and pepper.

3. Pour the dressing over the salad and toss to combine.

4. Refrigerate for at least 1 hour before serving to allow flavors to meld.

5. Serve chilled as a crunchy and satisfying side salad.

Nutrient:

Calories:	Fiber:	Protein:	Fat:
180	5g	6g	11g

Warm Brussels Sprouts Salad

Ingredients:

- 4 cups halved Brussels sprouts
- 1/4 cup chopped pecans, toasted
- 2 tablespoons dried cranberries
- 2 tablespoons olive oil
- 1 tablespoon balsamic vinegar
- 1 teaspoon Dijon mustard
- Salt and pepper to taste

1. Heat olive oil in a skillet over medium heat.

2. Add halved Brussels sprouts and cook for 8-10 minutes until tender and slightly caramelized.

3. In a small bowl, whisk together balsamic vinegar, Dijon mustard, salt, and pepper.

4. In a large bowl, combine cooked Brussels sprouts with chopped toasted pecans and dried cranberries.

5. Drizzle the dressing over the salad and toss to combine.

6. Serve warm as a hearty and flavorful side dish.

Nutrient :

Calories:	Fiber:	Protein:	Fat:
200	6g	5g	14g

Asian Edamame Salad

Ingredients:

- 2 cups shelled edamame, cooked
- 1 red bell pepper, thinly sliced
- 1 cup shredded red cabbage
- 1/4 cup chopped cilantro
- 2 tablespoons sesame oil
- 1 tablespoon rice vinegar
- 1 tablespoon soy sauce or tamari
- 1 tablespoon honey
- 1 teaspoon grated fresh ginger
- Salt and pepper to taste

Instructions:

1. In a large bowl, combine cooked shelled edamame, thinly sliced red bell pepper, shredded red cabbage, and chopped cilantro.

2. In a small bowl, whisk together sesame oil, rice vinegar, soy sauce or tamari, honey, grated fresh ginger, salt, and pepper.

3. Drizzle the dressing over the salad and toss to combine.

4. Serve chilled as a vibrant and protein-rich side salad.

Nutrient:

Calories:	Fiber:	Protein:	Fat:
220	8g	12g	10g

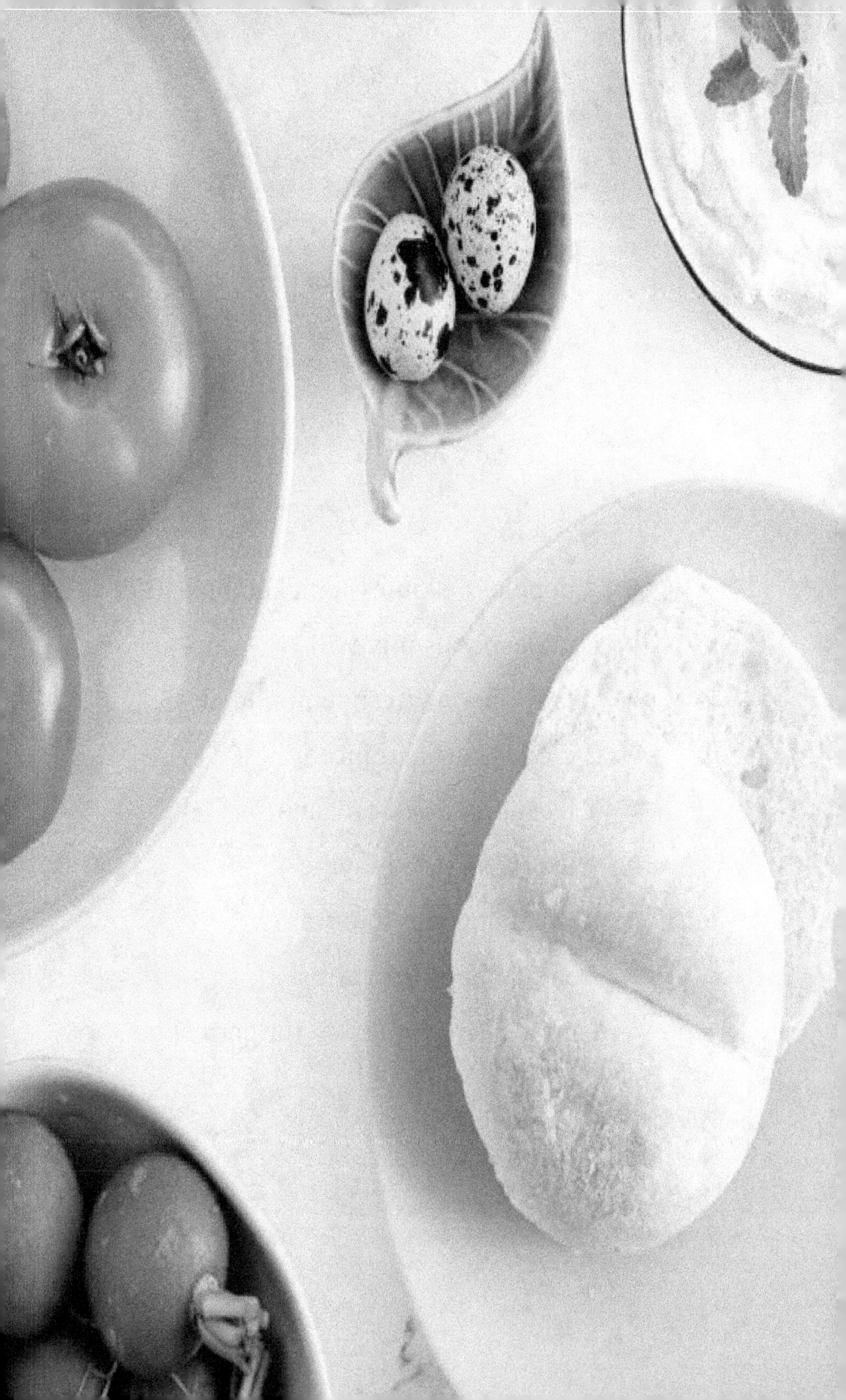

CHAPTER 5: MAIN COURSES: LIGHT AND NUTRITIOUS

Baked Lemon Herb Chicken

Ingredients:

- 4 boneless, skinless chicken breasts
- 2 tablespoons olive oil
- 2 tablespoons fresh lemon juice
- 2 cloves garlic, minced
- 1 teaspoon dried oregano
- 1 teaspoon dried thyme
- Salt and pepper to taste
- Lemon slices for garnish
- Chopped fresh parsley for garnish

1. Preheat the oven to 400°F (200°C).

2. In a bowl, whisk together olive oil, lemon juice, minced garlic, dried oregano, dried thyme, salt, and pepper.

3. Place chicken breasts in a baking dish and pour the marinade over them, turning to coat evenly.

4. Bake for 20-25 minutes until chicken is cooked through and juices run clear.

5. Garnish with lemon slices and chopped fresh parsley.

6. Serve hot with a side of steamed vegetables or quinoa.

Calories:	Protein	Carbohydrates:	Fat:
250	: 30g	2g	14g

Grilled Salmon with Dill Sauce

Ingredients:

- 4 salmon fillets
- 2 tablespoons olive oil
- Salt and pepper to taste
- Fresh dill, chopped
- 1/4 cup plain Greek yogurt
- 1 tablespoon lemon juice

Instructions:

1. Preheat the grill to medium-high heat.
2. Brush salmon fillets with olive oil and season with salt and pepper.

3. Grill salmon for 4-5 minutes per side until cooked through and flaky.

4. In a bowl, mix together chopped fresh dill, plain Greek yogurt, and lemon juice.

5. Serve grilled salmon with dill sauce drizzled on top.

6. Enjoy with a side of roasted vegetables or a green salad.

Nutrient:

✓ Calories: 300

✓ Protein: 25g

✓ Carbohydrates: 2g

✓ Fat: 20g

Turkey Meatballs with Marinara Sauce

Ingredients:

- 1 lb ground turkey
- 1/2 cup breadcrumbs (gluten-free if desired)
- 1/4 cup grated Parmesan cheese
- 1 egg, beaten
- 2 cloves garlic, minced
- 1 teaspoon dried oregano
- Salt and pepper to taste
- 2 cups marinara sauce (low-sodium)
- Fresh basil leaves for garnish

Instructions:

1. Preheat the oven to 400°F (200°C).
2. In a bowl, combine ground turkey, breadcrumbs, grated Parmesan

cheese, beaten egg, minced garlic, dried oregano, salt, and pepper.

3. Shape the mixture into meatballs and place on a baking sheet lined with parchment paper.

4. Bake meatballs for 20-25 minutes until cooked through.

5. Heat marinara sauce in a saucepan over medium heat.

6. Add cooked meatballs to the marinara sauce and simmer for 5-10 minutes.

7. Serve turkey meatballs with marinara sauce, garnished with fresh basil leaves.

8. Enjoy with whole-grain pasta or zucchini noodles.

- ✓ Calories: 280
- ✓ Protein: 25g
- ✓ Carbohydrates: 10g
- ✓ Fat: 15g

Lemon Garlic Shrimp Stir-Fry

Ingredients:

- 1 lb large shrimp, peeled and deveined
- 2 tablespoons olive oil
- 3 cloves garlic, minced
- 1 teaspoon grated fresh ginger
- 1 red bell pepper, sliced
- 1 cup snow peas
- 2 tablespoons low-sodium soy sauce or tamari
- Juice of 1 lemon
- Salt and pepper to taste

- Chopped green onions for garnish

Instructions:

1. Heat olive oil in a large skillet or wok over medium-high heat.

2. Add minced garlic and grated ginger, sauté for 1 minute until fragrant.

3. Add sliced red bell pepper and snow peas, stir-fry for 3-4 minutes until vegetables are tender-crisp.

4. Push vegetables to the side of the skillet and add shrimp to the center.

5. Cook shrimp for 2-3 minutes until pink and opaque.

6. Stir in low-sodium soy sauce or tamari, lemon juice, salt, and pepper.

7. Combine shrimp and vegetables, tossing to coat evenly.

8. Garnish with chopped green onions.

9. Serve hot over brown rice or cauliflower rice.

✓ Calories: 220

✓ Protein: 25g

✓ Carbohydrates: 8g

✓ Fat: 10g

Baked Cod with Herbed Quinoa

Ingredients:

- 4 cod fillets
- 2 tablespoons olive oil
- 2 cloves garlic, minced
- 1 tablespoon chopped fresh parsley
- 1 tablespoon chopped fresh dill
- Salt and pepper to taste
- 1 cup cooked quinoa

1. Preheat the oven to 400°F (200°C).

2. Place cod fillets in a baking dish lined with parchment paper.

3. In a bowl, combine olive oil, minced garlic, chopped fresh parsley, chopped fresh dill, salt, and pepper.

4. Brush the herb mixture over the cod fillets.

5. Bake for 15-20 minutes until fish is cooked through and flakes easily with a fork.

6. Serve baked cod over cooked quinoa.

7. Enjoy with a side of steamed broccoli or roasted vegetables.

Nutrient:

✓ Calories: 280

- ✓ Protein: 30g
- ✓ Carbohydrates: 12g
- ✓ Fat: 12g

Stuffed Bell Peppers with Ground Turkey

Ingredients:

- 4 bell peppers, tops cut off and seeds removed
- 1 lb ground turkey
- 1 cup cooked quinoa
- 1 can (14 oz) diced tomatoes, drained
- 1/2 cup chopped onion
- 2 cloves garlic, minced
- 1 teaspoon dried Italian seasoning
- Salt and pepper to taste
- 1/2 cup shredded mozzarella cheese

Instructions:

1. Preheat the oven to 375°F (190°C).

2. In a skillet, cook ground turkey, chopped onion, and minced garlic until turkey is browned.

3. Stir in cooked quinoa, diced tomatoes, dried Italian seasoning, salt, and pepper.

4. Spoon turkey mixture into hollowed-out bell peppers.

5. Place stuffed bell peppers in a baking dish.

6. Cover with foil and bake for 25-30 minutes until peppers are tender.

7. Remove foil, sprinkle shredded mozzarella cheese on top of each pepper, and bake uncovered for 5 more minutes until cheese is melted.

8. Serve stuffed bell peppers hot as a satisfying and colorful main course.

- ✓ Calories: 300
- ✓ Protein: 25g
- ✓ Carbohydrates: 20g
- ✓ Fat: 12g

Vegetarian Lentil Chili

Ingredients:

- 1 cup dry green lentils, rinsed
- 1 onion, chopped
- 2 cloves garlic, minced
- 1 red bell pepper, chopped
- 1 carrot, diced
- 1 zucchini, diced
- 1 can (14 oz) diced tomatoes
- 1 can (14 oz) kidney beans, drained and rinsed
- 1 tablespoon chili powder
- 1 teaspoon ground cumin

- Salt and pepper to taste
- Chopped fresh cilantro for garnish

Instructions:

1. In a large pot, combine dry green lentils with 3 cups of water.
2. Bring to a boil, then reduce heat and simmer for 15-20 minutes until lentils are tender.
3. In a separate skillet, sauté chopped onion and minced garlic until translucent.
4. Add chopped red bell pepper, diced carrot, and diced zucchini to the skillet, cooking for 5-7 minutes until vegetables are tender.
5. Add sautéed vegetables, diced tomatoes, kidney beans, chili powder, ground cumin, salt, and

pepper to the pot with cooked lentils.

6. Simmer chili for 15-20 minutes to allow flavors to meld.

7. Adjust seasoning if needed.

8. Serve vegetarian lentil chili hot, garnished with chopped fresh cilantro.

Nutrient:

✓ Calories: 280

✓ Protein: 18g

✓ Carbohydrates: 50g

✓ Fat: 2g

Eggplant Parmesan

Ingredients:

● 1 large eggplant, sliced into rounds

● 2 eggs, beaten

- 1 cup breadcrumbs (gluten-free if desired)
- 1/4 cup grated Parmesan cheese
- 2 cups marinara sauce (low-sodium)
- 1 cup shredded mozzarella cheese
- Fresh basil leaves for garnish

Instructions:

1. Preheat the oven to 400°F (200°C).
2. Dip eggplant slices into beaten eggs, then coat with breadcrumbs mixed with grated Parmesan cheese.
3. Place breaded eggplant slices on a baking sheet lined with parchment paper.
4. Bake for 20-25 minutes until eggplant is golden and crispy.
5. In a baking dish, spread a layer of marinara sauce.

6. Arrange baked eggplant slices over the marinara sauce.

7. Top eggplant slices with remaining marinara sauce and shredded mozzarella cheese.

8. Bake for an additional 15-20 minutes until cheese is melted and bubbly.

9. Garnish with fresh basil leaves.

10. Serve eggplant Parmesan hot as a comforting and satisfying main course.

Nutrient:

✓ Calories: 320

✓ Protein: 16g

✓ Carbohydrates: 30g

✓ Fat: 16g

Lemon Herb Baked Cod

Ingredients:

- 4 cod fillets
- 2 tablespoons olive oil
- 2 tablespoons fresh lemon juice
- 2 cloves garlic, minced
- 1 teaspoon dried thyme
- 1 teaspoon dried rosemary
- Salt and pepper to taste
- Lemon slices for garnish
- Chopped fresh parsley for garnish

Instructions:

1. Preheat the oven to 400°F (200°C).
2. In a bowl, whisk together olive oil, fresh lemon juice, minced garlic, dried thyme, dried rosemary, salt, and pepper.

3. Place cod fillets in a baking dish and pour the herb mixture over them, turning to coat evenly.

4. Arrange lemon slices on top of the cod fillets.

5. Bake for 15-20 minutes until fish is cooked through and flakes easily with a fork.

6. Garnish with chopped fresh parsley.

7. Serve hot with a side of steamed vegetables or quinoa.

Nutrient:

✓ Calories: 260

✓ Protein: 30g

✓ Carbohydrates: 2g

✓ Fat: 14g

Chicken Vegetable Stir-Fry

Ingredients:

- 2 boneless, skinless chicken breasts, thinly sliced
- 2 tablespoons olive oil
- 2 cloves garlic, minced
- 1-inch piece ginger, grated
- 1 red bell pepper, sliced
- 1 yellow bell pepper, sliced
- 1 cup broccoli florets
- 1 cup snow peas
- 2 tablespoons low-sodium soy sauce or tamari
- 1 tablespoon hoisin sauce (optional)
- Salt and pepper to taste
- Chopped green onions for garnish

1. Heat olive oil in a large skillet or wok over medium-high heat.

2. Add minced garlic and grated ginger, sauté for 1 minute until fragrant.

3. Add thinly sliced chicken breasts and cook for 4-5 minutes until browned and cooked through.

4. Add sliced red bell pepper, sliced yellow bell pepper, broccoli florets, and snow peas to the skillet.

5. Stir-fry vegetables for 3-4 minutes until tender-crisp.

6. Stir in low-sodium soy sauce or tamari and hoisin sauce (if using).

7. Season with salt and pepper to taste.

8. Garnish with chopped green onions.

9. Serve chicken vegetable stir-fry hot over brown rice or cauliflower rice.

Nutrient:

- ✓ Calories: 280
- ✓ Protein: 30g
- ✓ Carbohydrates: 12g
- ✓ Fat: 12g

CHAPTER 6: SNACKS AND SMALL BITES

Greek Yogurt Parfait

Ingredients:

- 1 cup plain Greek yogurt
- 1/2 cup fresh berries (e.g., strawberries, blueberries)
- 2 tablespoons chopped nuts (e.g., almonds, walnuts)
- 1 tablespoon honey (optional)

Instructions:

1. In a small bowl or glass, layer Greek yogurt, fresh berries, and chopped nuts.
2. Drizzle with honey if desired.
3. Serve immediately as a protein-rich and satisfying snack.

- ✓ Calories: 200
- ✓ Protein: 15g
- ✓ Carbohydrates: 20g
- ✓ Fat: 8g

Avocado Egg Salad Cucumber Bites

Ingredients:

- 2 hard-boiled eggs, peeled and mashed
- 1 ripe avocado, mashed
- 1 tablespoon Greek yogurt
- Salt and pepper to taste
- 1 English cucumber, sliced into rounds

1. In a bowl, combine mashed hard-boiled eggs, mashed avocado, Greek yogurt, salt, and pepper.
2. Place a dollop of avocado egg salad on each cucumber round.
3. Serve as a refreshing and nutritious finger food.

Nutrient:

- ✓ Calories: 120
- ✓ Protein: 6g
- ✓ Carbohydrates: 8g
- ✓ Fat: 8g

Hummus Stuffed Mini Peppers

Ingredients:

- 12 mini sweet peppers
- 1/2 cup hummus
- Fresh parsley or paprika for garnish

Instructions:

1. Slice the tops off the mini peppers and remove seeds.
2. Fill each mini pepper with hummus.
3. Garnish with fresh parsley or a sprinkle of paprika.
4. Serve chilled as a colorful and flavorful snack.

Nutrient:

- ✓ Calories: 80
- ✓ Protein: 3g
- ✓ Carbohydrates: 10g

✓ Fat: 4g

Cottage Cheese with Pineapple

Ingredients:

- 1/2 cup low-fat cottage cheese
- 1/2 cup fresh pineapple chunks

Instructions:

1. In a bowl, combine low-fat cottage cheese and fresh pineapple chunks.
2. Mix well.
3. Enjoy as a quick and protein-packed snack.

Nutrient:

✓ Protein: 15g

✓ Carbohydrates: 15g

✓ Fat: 3g

Smoked Salmon Cucumber Bites

Ingredients:

- 4 oz smoked salmon
- 1 cucumber, sliced into rounds
- 2 tablespoons cream cheese
- Fresh dill for garnish

Instructions:

1. Spread cream cheese on each cucumber round.
2. Top with smoked salmon.
3. Garnish with fresh dill.
4. Serve as elegant and satisfying finger food.

Nutrient:

- ✓ Calories: 120
- ✓ Protein: 12g
- ✓ Carbohydrates: 2g

✓ Fat: 7g

Almond Butter Banana Bites

Ingredients:

- 1 banana, sliced
- 2 tablespoons almond butter
- 2 tablespoons granola

Instructions:

1. Spread almond butter on banana slices.
2. Sprinkle with granola.
3. Serve immediately for a crunchy and nutritious snack.

Nutrient:

✓ Calories: 200

✓ Protein: 5g

✓ Carbohydrates: 25g

- ✓ Fat: 10g

Caprese Skewers

Ingredients:

- Cherry tomatoes
- Fresh mozzarella balls
- Fresh basil leaves
- Balsamic glaze (optional)

Instructions:

1. Thread cherry tomatoes, fresh mozzarella balls, and fresh basil leaves onto small skewers.
2. Drizzle with balsamic glaze if desired.
3. Serve as a delightful and colorful appetizer.

Nutrient:

- ✓ Calories: 120
- ✓ Protein: 6g

✓ Carbohydrates: 3g

✓ Fat: 9g

Apple Slices with Almond Butter

Ingredients:

- 1 apple, sliced
- 2 tablespoons almond butter

Instructions:

1. Spread almond butter on apple slices.

2. Serve as a satisfying and crunchy snack.

Nutrient:

✓ Calories: 200

✓ Protein: 4g

- ✓ Carbohydrates: 25g
- ✓ Fat: 10g

Stuffed Cherry Tomatoes

Ingredients:

- Cherry tomatoes
- 1/2 cup tuna salad (canned tuna mixed with Greek yogurt and chopped celery)

Instructions:

1. Cut the tops off cherry tomatoes and scoop out seeds.
2. Fill each cherry tomato with tuna salad.
3. Serve as a protein-rich and flavorful snack.

Nutrient:

- ✓ Calories: 80
- ✓ Protein: 8g
- ✓ Carbohydrates: 3g

✓ Fat: 4g

Greek Cucumber Cups

Ingredients:

- 2 large cucumbers
- 1/2 cup Greek yogurt
- 1/4 cup chopped black olives
- 1/4 cup diced cucumber
- 1 tablespoon chopped fresh dill
- Salt and pepper to taste

Instructions:

1. Peel strips of cucumber skin lengthwise, leaving some skin intact for a striped effect.

2. Cut cucumbers into thick rounds and hollow out the centers to create cups.

3. In a bowl, mix Greek yogurt, chopped black olives, diced

cucumber, chopped fresh dill, salt, and pepper.

4. Fill cucumber cups with Greek yogurt mixture.

5. Serve chilled as a refreshing and savory snack.

Nutrient:

✓ Calories: 80

✓ Protein: 5g

✓ Carbohydrates: 7g

✓ Fat: 4g

Zucchini Fritters

Ingredients:

- 2 medium zucchini, grated

- 1/4 cup almond flour or gluten-free breadcrumbs

- 2 eggs

- 1/4 cup grated Parmesan cheese
- 2 tablespoons chopped fresh parsley
- Salt and pepper to taste
- Olive oil for frying

Instructions:

1. Place grated zucchini in a clean kitchen towel and squeeze out excess moisture.
2. In a bowl, combine grated zucchini, almond flour or breadcrumbs, eggs, grated Parmesan cheese, chopped fresh parsley, salt, and pepper.
3. Heat olive oil in a skillet over medium heat.
4. Drop spoonfuls of zucchini mixture into the skillet, flattening slightly to form fritters.
5. Cook for 3-4 minutes per side until golden and crispy.

6. Drain on paper towels.

7. Serve zucchini fritters warm with a dollop of Greek yogurt or a squeeze of lemon.

- ✓ Calories: 150
- ✓ Protein: 8g
- ✓ Carbohydrates: 6g
- ✓ Fat: 10g

Stuffed Mushrooms

Ingredients:

- 12 large button mushrooms
- 1/2 cup cooked quinoa
- 1/4 cup chopped spinach
- 2 tablespoons chopped sun-dried tomatoes

- 2 tablespoons grated Parmesan cheese
- 1 tablespoon olive oil
- Salt and pepper to taste

Instructions:

1. Preheat the oven to 375°F (190°C).

2. Remove stems from mushrooms and chop finely.

3. In a bowl, combine chopped mushroom stems, cooked quinoa, chopped spinach, chopped sun-dried tomatoes, grated Parmesan cheese, olive oil, salt, and pepper.

4. Stuff mushroom caps with quinoa mixture.

5. Place stuffed mushrooms on a baking sheet.

6. Bake for 15-20 minutes until mushrooms are tender and filling is heated through.

7. Serve stuffed mushrooms warm as a savory appetizer or snack.

Nutrient:

- ✓ Calories: 120
- ✓ Protein: 6g
- ✓ Carbohydrates: 10g
- ✓ Fat: 6g

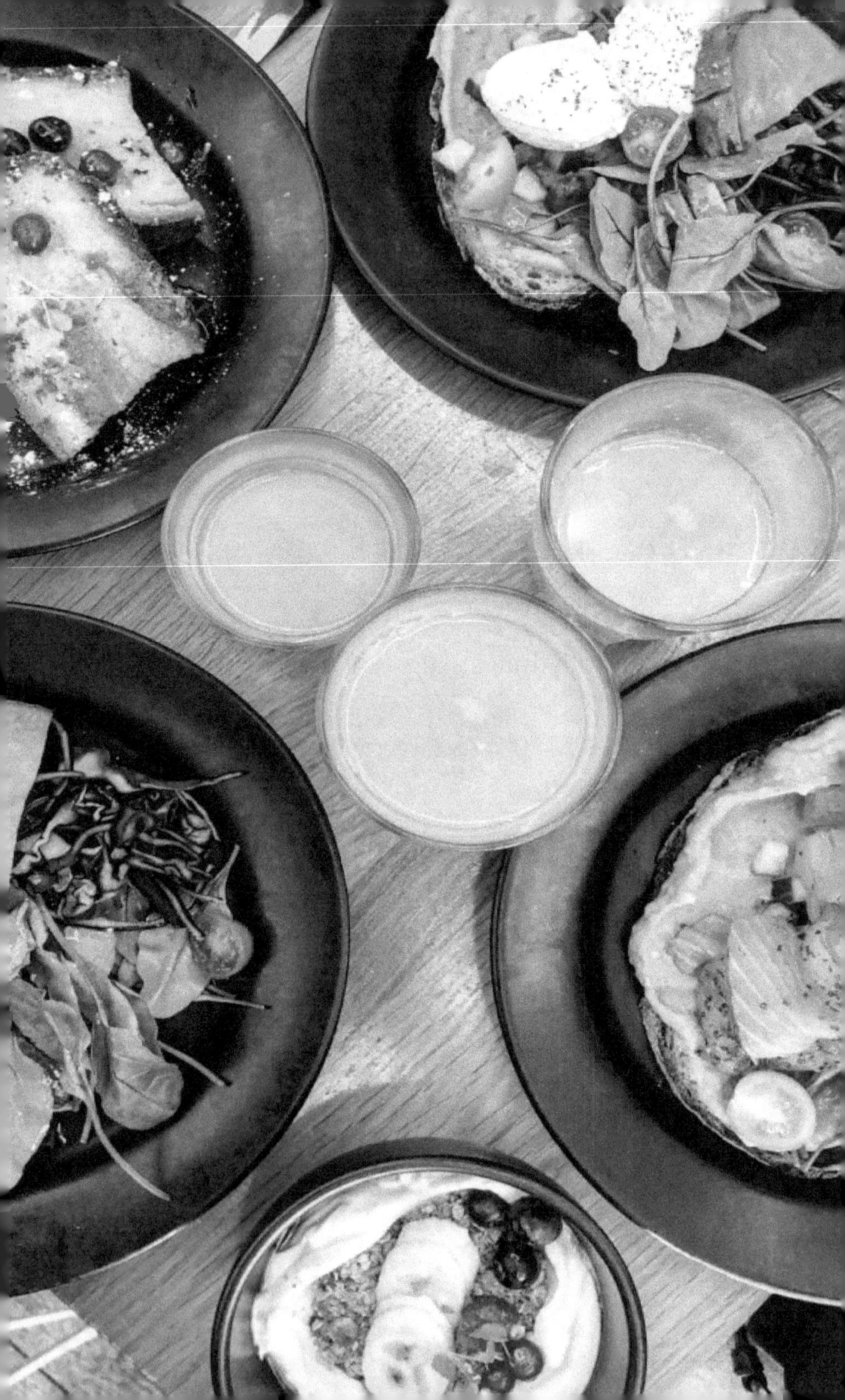

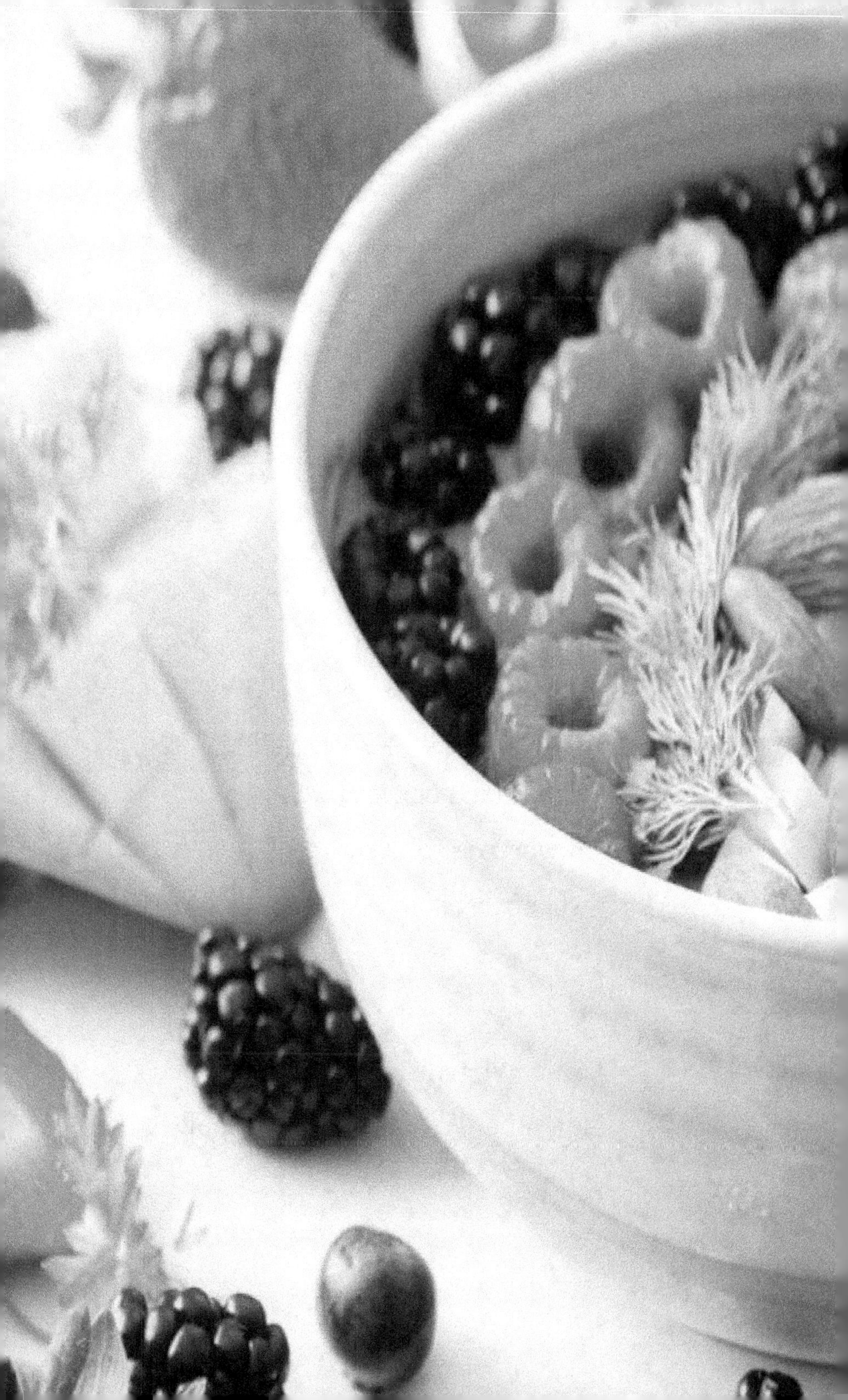

CHAPTER 7: DESSERTS AND TREATS

Mixed Berry Chia Seed Pudding

Ingredients:

- 1/4 cup chia seeds
- 1 cup unsweetened almond milk
- 1 tablespoon honey or maple syrup
- 1 cup mixed berries (e.g., strawberries, blueberries, raspberries)

Instructions:

1. In a bowl, whisk together chia seeds, almond milk, and honey or maple syrup.

2. Let the mixture sit for 10 minutes,
   then stir again to prevent clumping.

3. Refrigerate for at least 2 hours or
   overnight until thickened.

4. Layer chia seed pudding with
   mixed berries in serving glasses.

5. Serve chilled as a nutritious and
   fiber-rich dessert.

Nutrient:

- ✓ Calories: 180
- ✓ Protein: 5g
- ✓ Carbohydrates: 25g
- ✓ Fat: 7g

Baked Apples with Cinnamon and Walnuts

Ingredients:

- 4 apples, cored
- 2 tablespoons chopped walnuts

- 1 tablespoon honey
- 1 teaspoon ground cinnamon

Instructions:

1. Preheat the oven to 375°F (190°C).

2. Place cored apples in a baking dish.

3. In a bowl, mix chopped walnuts, honey, and ground cinnamon.

4. Stuff each apple with the walnut mixture.

5. Bake for 25-30 minutes until apples are tender.

6. Serve baked apples warm as a comforting and naturally sweet dessert.

Nutrient:

- ✓ Calories: 150
- ✓ Protein: 2g
- ✓ Carbohydrates: 30g

✓ Fat: 4g

Greek Yogurt Popsicles

Ingredients:

- 1 cup plain Greek yogurt
- 1 cup mixed berries (e.g., strawberries, blueberries)
- 2 tablespoons honey or maple syrup

Instructions:

1. In a blender, combine Greek yogurt, mixed berries, and honey or maple syrup.
2. Blend until smooth.
3. Pour mixture into popsicle molds.
4. Insert popsicle sticks and freeze for at least 4 hours until solid.

5. Unmold Greek yogurt popsicles and enjoy as a refreshing and protein-rich treat.

Nutrient:

- ✓ Calories: 120
- ✓ Protein: 8g
- ✓ Carbohydrates: 20g
- ✓ Fat: 2g

Banana Oat Cookies

Ingredients:

- 2 ripe bananas, mashed
- 1 cup rolled oats
- 1/4 cup chopped walnuts or raisins
- 1 teaspoon ground cinnamon

1. Preheat the oven to 350°F (175°C).

2. In a bowl, combine mashed bananas, rolled oats, chopped walnuts or raisins, and ground cinnamon.

3. Drop spoonfuls of the mixture onto a baking sheet lined with parchment paper.

4. Flatten each spoonful with the back of a fork.

5. Bake for 15-20 minutes until cookies are golden.

6. Let cool before serving.

Nutrient:

✓ Calories: 90

✓ Protein: 2g

✓ Carbohydrates: 18g

✓ Fat: 2g

Coconut Chia Pudding

Ingredients:

- 1/4 cup chia seeds
- 1 cup coconut milk
- 2 tablespoons shredded coconut
- 1 tablespoon honey or maple syrup
- Fresh mango slices for garnish

Instructions:

1. In a bowl, whisk together chia seeds, coconut milk, shredded coconut, and honey or maple syrup.

2. Let the mixture sit for 10 minutes, then stir again to prevent clumping.

3. Refrigerate for at least 2 hours or overnight until thickened.

4. Serve coconut chia pudding in dessert bowls, garnished with fresh mango slices.

- ✓ Calories: 220
- ✓ Protein: 5g
- ✓ Carbohydrates: 20g
- ✓ Fat: 15g

Chocolate Avocado Mousse

Ingredients:

- 2 ripe avocados
- 1/4 cup cocoa powder
- 1/4 cup honey or maple syrup
- 1 teaspoon vanilla extract
- Pinch of salt
- Fresh berries for garnish

Instructions:

1. In a food processor, combine ripe avocados, cocoa powder, honey or maple syrup, vanilla extract, and salt.
2. Blend until smooth and creamy.

3. Spoon chocolate avocado mousse into serving bowls.

4. Chill for at least 30 minutes before serving.

5. Garnish with fresh berries.

✓ Calories: 200

✓ Protein: 3g

✓ Carbohydrates: 20g

✓ Fat: 14g

Frozen Yogurt Bark

Ingredients:

- 2 cups plain Greek yogurt
- 1/4 cup honey or maple syrup
- 1/2 cup mixed berries (e.g., strawberries, blueberries)
- 1/4 cup chopped nuts (e.g., almonds, pecans)

Instructions:

1. In a bowl, mix Greek yogurt and honey or maple syrup.

2. Spread yogurt mixture evenly on a baking sheet lined with parchment paper.

3. Sprinkle mixed berries and chopped nuts over the yogurt.

4. Freeze for 2-3 hours until firm.

5. Break frozen yogurt bark into pieces and enjoy as a refreshing and crunchy dessert.

Nutrient:

- ✓ Calories: 150
- ✓ Protein: 8g
- ✓ Carbohydrates: 20g
- ✓ Fat: 5g

Pumpkin Spice Energy Bites

Ingredients:

- 1 cup rolled oats
- 1/2 cup pumpkin puree
- 1/4 cup almond butter
- 2 tablespoons honey or maple syrup
- 1 teaspoon pumpkin pie spice
- 1/4 cup mini chocolate chips (optional)

Instructions:

1. In a bowl, mix rolled oats, pumpkin puree, almond butter, honey or maple syrup, pumpkin pie spice, and mini chocolate chips.

2. Roll mixture into small balls using your hands.

3. Refrigerate for at least 1 hour to firm up.

4. Serve pumpkin spice energy bites chilled as a satisfying and flavorful snack.

Nutrient:

- ✓ Calories: 120
- ✓ Protein: 3g
- ✓ Carbohydrates: 15g
- ✓ Fat: 6g

Berry Frozen Yogurt Cups

Ingredients:

- 2 cups plain Greek yogurt
- 1 cup mixed berries (e.g., strawberries, blueberries)
- 2 tablespoons honey or maple syrup
- 1/4 cup granola

Instructions:

1. In a blender, combine Greek yogurt, mixed berries, and honey or maple syrup.

2. Blend until smooth.

3. Spoon mixture into muffin tin cups lined with paper liners.

4. Top each cup with granola.

5. Freeze for 4 hours until set.

6. Remove frozen yogurt cups from muffin tin and peel off paper liners before serving.

Nutrient:

✓ Calories: 150

✓ Protein: 8g

✓ Carbohydrates: 20g

✓ Fat: 4g

Lemon Coconut Bliss Balls

- 1 cup shredded coconut
- Zest and juice of 1 lemon
- 1/4 cup almond flour
- 2 tablespoons honey or maple syrup
- 2 tablespoons coconut oil, melted

Instructions:

1. In a bowl, combine shredded coconut, lemon zest, almond flour, honey or maple syrup, and melted coconut oil.
2. Mix until well combined and sticky.
3. Roll mixture into small balls using your hands.
4. Refrigerate for 30 minutes to firm up.

5. Serve lemon coconut bliss balls chilled as a zesty and delightful dessert.

- ✓ Calories: 120
- ✓ Protein: 2g
- ✓ Carbohydrates: 10g
- ✓ Fat: 9g

Almond Flour Banana Bread

Ingredients:

- 2 ripe bananas, mashed
- 2 eggs
- 1/4 cup coconut oil, melted
- 1/4 cup honey or maple syrup
- 1 teaspoon vanilla extract
- 2 cups almond flour
- 1/2 teaspoon baking soda

- Pinch of salt
- Optional: chopped nuts or dark chocolate chips

Instructions:

1. Preheat the oven to 350°F (175°C). Grease a loaf pan with coconut oil.
2. In a bowl, whisk together mashed bananas, eggs, melted coconut oil, honey or maple syrup, and vanilla extract.
3. Add almond flour, baking soda, and salt. Mix until well combined.
4. Fold in chopped nuts or dark chocolate chips if using.
5. Pour batter into the prepared loaf pan.
6. Bake for 45-50 minutes until golden and a toothpick inserted into the center comes out clean.

7. Let banana bread cool before slicing.

Nutrient:

- ✓ Calories: 180
- ✓ Protein: 5g
- ✓ Carbohydrates: 15g
- ✓ Fat: 12g

Chia Coconut Mango Popsicles

- Ingredients:
- 1 cup coconut milk
- 2 tablespoons chia seeds
- 2 tablespoons honey or maple syrup
- 1 ripe mango, peeled and diced

Instructions:

1. In a bowl, whisk together coconut milk, chia seeds, and honey or maple syrup.

2. Let the mixture sit for 10 minutes, then stir again to prevent clumping.

3. Stir in diced mango.

4. Pour mixture into popsicle molds.

5. Insert popsicle sticks and freeze for at least 4 hours until solid.

6. Unmold chia coconut mango popsicles and enjoy as a tropical and refreshing dessert.

Nutrient:

✓ Calories: 120

✓ Protein: 3g

✓ Carbohydrates: 20g

✓ Fat: 4g

CHAPTER 8:

BEVERAGES FOR

DIGESTIVE COMFORT

Ginger Turmeric Tea

Ingredients:

- 1-inch piece of fresh ginger, sliced
- 1 teaspoon ground turmeric
- 2 cups water
- Honey (optional, to taste)
- Lemon slices (optional)

Instructions:

1. In a small saucepan, combine sliced ginger, ground turmeric, and water.
2. Bring to a simmer over medium heat.

3. Reduce heat and let it simmer for 5-7 minutes.

4. Strain the tea into mugs.

5. Sweeten with honey if desired and garnish with lemon slices.

6. Serve warm and enjoy the soothing benefits of ginger and turmeric.

Nutrient:

✓ Calories: 10

✓ Carbohydrates: 2g

✓ Fat: 0g

✓ Protein: 0g

Peppermint Infusion

Ingredients:

- 1 tablespoon dried peppermint leaves (or 3-4 fresh peppermint sprigs)
- 2 cups boiling water
- Honey (optional, to taste)

Instructions:

1. Place dried peppermint leaves or fresh peppermint sprigs in a teapot or heatproof pitcher.
2. Pour boiling water over the peppermint.
3. Cover and steep for 5-7 minutes.
4. Strain the infusion into mugs.
5. Sweeten with honey if desired.
6. Serve warm for a refreshing and digestive-soothing drink.

Nutrient:

- ✓ Calories: 5
- ✓ Carbohydrates: 1g
- ✓ Fat: 0g
- ✓ Protein: 0g

Chamomile and Lemon Balm Tea

Ingredients:

- 1 tablespoon dried chamomile flowers
- 1 tablespoon dried lemon balm leaves
- 2 cups boiling water
- Honey (optional, to taste)
- Lemon slices (optional)

Instructions:

1. Combine dried chamomile flowers and dried lemon balm leaves in a teapot or heatproof pitcher.
2. Pour boiling water over the herbs.
3. Cover and steep for 5-10 minutes.
4. Strain the tea into mugs.
5. Sweeten with honey if desired and garnish with lemon slices.
6. Serve warm as a calming and stomach-soothing beverage.

Nutrient:

✓ Calories: 5
✓ Carbohydrates: 1g
✓ Fat: 0g
✓ Protein: 0g

Aloe Vera Juice Refresher

- 1/4 cup pure aloe vera juice
- 1 cup coconut water or plain water
- 1 tablespoon fresh lemon juice
- 1 teaspoon honey (optional)

Instructions:

1. In a glass, mix together aloe vera juice, coconut water or plain water, and fresh lemon juice.
2. Sweeten with honey if desired.
3. Stir well until combined.
4. Serve chilled over ice for a hydrating and soothing beverage.

Nutrient:

- ✓ Calories: 30
- ✓ Carbohydrates: 8g
- ✓ Fat: 0g

✓ Protein: 0g

Ingredients:

- 1 cup fresh pineapple chunks
- 1-inch piece of fresh ginger, peeled
- 1/2 cup plain Greek yogurt
- 1/2 cup coconut water or plain water
- Ice cubes (optional)

Instructions:

1. In a blender, combine fresh pineapple chunks, peeled ginger, plain Greek yogurt, and coconut water or plain water.
2. Blend until smooth.
3. Add ice cubes if desired for a chilled smoothie.

4. Pour into glasses and enjoy this refreshing and digestion-friendly smoothie.

✓ Calories: 120

✓ Carbohydrates: 20g

✓ Fat: 1g

✓ Protein: 8g

Cucumber Mint Cooler

Ingredients:

● 1 cucumber, peeled and sliced

● Handful of fresh mint leaves

● Juice of 1 lime

● 2 cups cold water

● Stevia or honey (optional, to taste)

1. In a blender, combine cucumber slices, fresh mint leaves, lime juice, and cold water.
2. Blend until smooth.
3. Sweeten with stevia or honey if desired.
4. Strain the mixture into a pitcher to remove any pulp.
5. Serve chilled over ice for a refreshing and hydrating drink.

Nutrient:

✓ Calories: 15
✓ Carbohydrates: 4g
✓ Fat: 0g
✓ Protein: 1g

Banana Almond Smoothie

Ingredients:

- 1 ripe banana
- 1 tablespoon almond butter
- 1 cup almond milk
- 1 tablespoon ground flaxseeds
- Pinch of ground cinnamon

Instructions:

1. In a blender, combine ripe banana, almond butter, almond milk, ground flaxseeds, and ground cinnamon.
2. Blend until smooth and creamy.
3. Pour into glasses and enjoy this nutrient-packed and easy-to-digest smoothie.

- ✓ Calories: 200
- ✓ Carbohydrates: 30g
- ✓ Fat: 8g
- ✓ Protein: 5g

Green Tea with Lemon

Ingredients:

- 1 green tea bag
- 1 cup hot water
- Squeeze of fresh lemon juice
- Stevia or honey (optional, to taste)

Instructions:

1. Place a green tea bag in a mug and pour hot water over it.
2. Let it steep for 3-5 minutes.
3. Remove the tea bag and squeeze in fresh lemon juice.

4. Sweeten with stevia or honey if desired.

5. Stir well and enjoy this antioxidant-rich and refreshing beverage.

✓ Calories: 0

✓ Carbohydrates: 0g

✓ Fat: 0g

✓ Protein: 0g

Warm Lemon Water

Ingredients:

● Juice of 1/2 lemon

● 1 cup warm water

1. Squeeze the juice of half a lemon into a cup of warm water.
2. Stir well.
3. Drink first thing in the morning on an empty stomach for gentle detoxification and digestive support.

Nutrient:

✓ Calories: 5

✓ Carbohydrates: 2g

✓ Fat: 0g

✓ Protein: 0g

Herbal Infusion with Fennel and Coriander

Ingredients:

- 1 teaspoon fennel seeds
- 1 teaspoon coriander seeds
- 2 cups boiling water

- Honey (optional, to taste)

Instructions:

1. In a teapot or heatproof pitcher, combine fennel seeds and coriander seeds.
2. Pour boiling water over the seeds.
3. Cover and steep for 10-15 minutes.
4. Strain the infusion into mugs.
5. Sweeten with honey if desired.
6. Enjoy this herbal infusion for its digestive benefits.

Nutrient:

✓ Calories: 5
✓ Carbohydrates: 1g
✓ Fat: 0g
✓ Protein: 0g

Golden Milk (Turmeric Latte)

Ingredients:

- 1 cup unsweetened almond milk
- 1/2 teaspoon ground turmeric
- 1/4 teaspoon ground cinnamon
- Pinch of ground black pepper
- 1 teaspoon honey or maple syrup (optional)

Instructions:

1. In a small saucepan, heat almond milk over medium-low heat.
2. Whisk in ground turmeric, ground cinnamon, and ground black pepper.
3. Add honey or maple syrup if desired for sweetness.
4. Heat until warm but not boiling.

5. Pour into a mug and enjoy this comforting and anti-inflammatory beverage.

✓ Calories: 40

✓ Carbohydrates: 3g

✓ Fat: 3g

✓ Protein: 1g

Papaya and Pineapple Smoothie

Ingredients:

- 1/2 cup fresh papaya chunks
- 1/2 cup fresh pineapple chunks
- 1/2 cup coconut water or plain water
- 1 tablespoon fresh lime juice
- Ice cubes (optional)

1. In a blender, combine fresh papaya chunks, fresh pineapple chunks, coconut water or plain water, and fresh lime juice.
2. Blend until smooth.
3. Add ice cubes if desired for a refreshing and tropical smoothie.
4. Pour into glasses and enjoy this hydrating and digestion-friendly beverage.

Nutrient:

- ✓ Calories: 70
- ✓ Carbohydrates: 18g
- ✓ Fat: 0g
- ✓ Protein: 1g

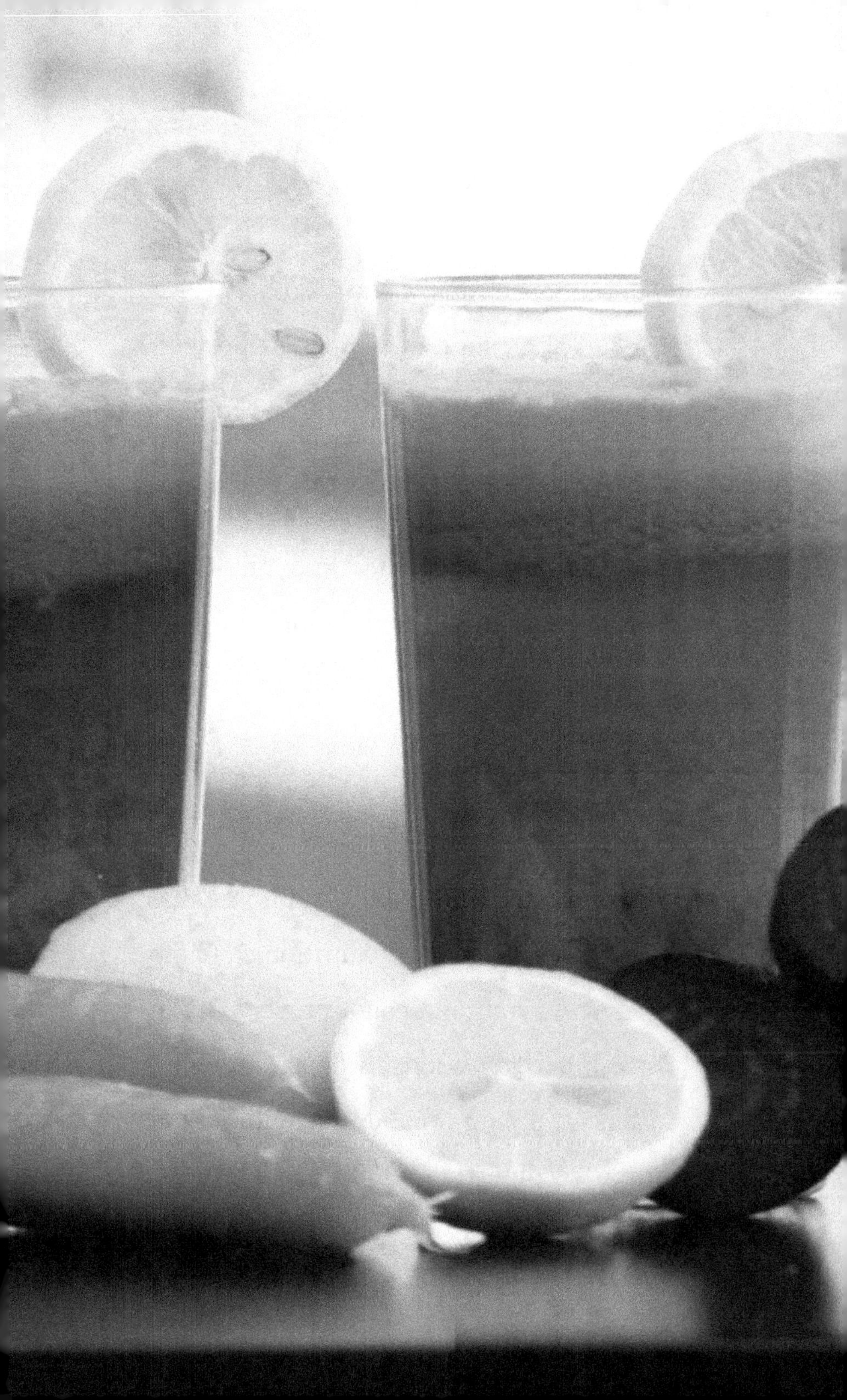

CONCLUSION

Throughout this cookbook, we've looked at a range of recipes made with diverticulitis in mind. From breakfast to main dishes, soups, salads, snacks, and desserts, each cuisine is designed to be easy on the stomach while providing important nutrients and flavors.

Understanding diverticulitis is essential for making informed dietary decisions.

We've talked about the condition, what it comprises, and how nutrition can help manage symptoms and prevent flare-ups. Fiber-rich foods, proper water, and attentive eating practices can all greatly improve digestive comfort and general well-being.

Fiber plays an essential part in a diverticulitis-friendly diet. Fiber regulates bowel motions, maintains gut health, and encourages the growth of good bacteria in the colon. Fiber-rich foods such as fruits, vegetables, whole grains, and legumes can help with digestion and minimize the risk of problems.

Fluid intake is another important part of digestive health, since it keeps stools soft and helps with bowel motions.

This cookbook includes hydrating beverages and refreshing smoothies that promote general hydration and intestinal comfort.